NO CH

For every woman, I hope
that she no longer, unless s
off during the menopause with prescriptions for palliatives such as aspirin, Librium or Valium, or worse still
dismissed with the words, 'It's just your age. There is
nothing to be done. You must put up with it.'
There is a great deal to be done. You don't have to put
up with it. The choice is *yours*.

Wendy Cooper

Also by Wendy Cooper

Understanding Osteoporosis
The Fertile Years
Everything you need to know about the Pill
Human Potential

Wendy Cooper

No Change

HRT – A biological revolution for women

ARROW

*'Though her years were waving,
her climacteric teased her
like her "teens".'*

– *Lord Bryon, Don Juan*

This edition published by Arrow Books in 1996

1 3 5 7 9 10 8 6 4 2

© Wendy Cooper 1975

The right of Wendy Cooper to be identified as the author
of this work has been asserted by her in accordance
with the Copyright, Designs and Patents Act, 1988

First published in the United Kingdom in 1975 by
Hutchinson

Arrow Books Limited
Random House UK Ltd,
20 Vauxhall Bridge Road, London SW1V 2SA

Random House Australia (Pty) Limited
16 Dalmore Drive, Scoresby
Victoria 3179, Australia

Random House New Zealand Limited
18 Poland Road, Glenfield
Auckland 10, New Zealand

Random House South Africa (Pty) Limited
PO Box 2263, Rosebank 2121, South Africa

Random House UK Limited Reg. No. 954009

A CIP catalogue record for this book
is available from the British Library

Papers used by Random House UK Limited
are natural, recyclable products made from wood grown in
sustainable forests. The manufacturing processes conform to the
environmental regulations of the country of origin.

ISBN 0 09 922812 2

Phototypeset by Intype London Ltd

Printed and bound in Great Britain by
Cox & Wyman Ltd, Reading, Berkshire

Contents

Foreword

by Sir John Peel KCVO FRCP FRCS

I am pleased to write a brief foreword to Wendy Cooper's book on the menopause, because, having read it with ease and interest, I am sure it will help a great many women who read it to have a better understanding of the many problems relating to their physical and mental health which occur at this particular time of their lives. Being written by a laywoman, it is in a language and style more easily understood and appreciated by a lay reader. The author has taken a quite remarkable amount of time and trouble to inform herself about the subject. She has visited clinics and specialists in Europe and North America as well as in Britain; she has spent hours on the telephone talking to doctors and victims, and shown a monumental degree of patience in reading letters received and in answering them. She has obtained the personal views of many gynaecologists and physicians, and faithfully recorded them and delved with unusual dedication into the literature.

The changes that affect both the body and the mind at and after the menopause are immensely complicated. Not only are there hormonal changes, but also emotional, social and family changes, and no one really knows why in fact some women, albeit the minority, pass through their fifties and sixties with little physical or emotional disturbance.

I am convinced from experience that Hormone Replacement Therapy can be of immense help to a great many women, but I am equally certain that it should only be made available under very strict medical supervision. Not only do we not know all about the biochemical interactions that take place when Oestrogen Replacement Therapy is given but we certainly do not know all the long-term side-effects.

If Wendy Cooper's book is widely read, as I hope it will be, it should do much to educate women about themselves and to stimulate them to seek medical advice instead of putting up with unpleasant and at times disastrous symptoms in the belief that they are the inevitable consequences of being a woman who must grin and bear it all.

The author's enthusiasm and dedication emerge from every page of the book, and if this leads her to over-simplification and even exaggeration at times this is no bad thing; such is the path the pioneer must tread. I wish this book every success.

Author's Note (1996)

The above foreword was written by Sir John Peel to introduce the very first edition of this book in 1975. I believe it still gives women confidence to know that the Queen's gynaecologist was already using HRT for menopause patients at a time when other, less well informed, still deemed it too controversial. His public support in those early days did much to establish medical respectability for this treatment and to speed the process of research here.

Since then Sir John has seen the work carried out in our British Menopause Clinics resolving many of the questions about long term safety which he rightly felt needed further study. In particular it has confirmed the wisdom and value of the 'combined' form of HRT, which he himself had always advocated and so strongly endorses in this book.

Each new edition of *No Change* has recorded the progress of this British work in appropriate sections of the text, but fuller information on this is given in Appendix 3, together with details of new, simple tests for early diagnosis of osteoporosis and of any further developments in HRT as we go to press.

This edition can also record belated but significant official recognition of the value and importance of Hormone Replacement Therapy. Following the special report in 1989 by the Royal College of Physicians, sent to all GPs and advocating wider usage of HRT, in 1995 the Department of Health issued similar recommendations, directed to local health authorities in particular, urging better facilities for detection and treatment of osteoporosis.

It has taken nearly a quarter of a century, but at last HRT has come in from the cold. This is the story of the struggle and the victory, but above all of what HRT can do for you.

Wendy Cooper
September 1996

Introduction – The choice is yours

Just once or twice in the life of a working journalist, there comes a story so exciting, important and demanding that it refuses to be written out or written off. You may present it in a dozen different ways for a dozen different papers and magazines. In the process *you* may become exhausted, but the subject does not. Instead of public interest and response declining, they increase. The law of diminishing returns fails to operate. In the end you have to recognize that instead of *you* running the story, the story is running you.

It has been that way for me with the story of Hormone Replacement Therapy (HRT) to eliminate the menopause. This revolutionary medical concept sees the menopause as a hormone deficiency condition, and sets out to treat it by replacing the declining oestrogen. In 1971 I began intensive research both here and in America and in 1973 I published the first series of articles entitled 'A Change for the Better' in the *London Evening News*. Ever since then there has been a continuous demand for major features on the same subject, for radio and television programmes and for talks; not just talks to women either, but sometimes, and surprisingly, to doctors.

Even when I have turned to other subjects, these have tended to be related, arising out of different aspects of the same research, and so HRT (by now we are on familiar terms) still found its way legitimately into several more general features on ageing. But it also insinuated itself far less predictably into features on show business ladies, on Women's Lib and even into a serious study on the status of women.

But HRT not only began to take over my professional life, it took over at home too, invading it with a vast physical presence. The files of reports, surveys and medical papers (still growing) proved too bulky to stand on the shelves in my study and spilled over to cover every flat surface. But the file of which I was always most conscious, which seemed to sit there in mute reproach, was the one containing the letters I have received from women – over five thousand of them.

These letters made two things uncomfortably clear. Firstly, that despite the complacent attitude of many doctors, who at that time were insisting that the menopause was only a temporary inconvenience and nothing to make a fuss about, there were, in fact, many women who suffered from it both acutely and for a long time. Secondly they made clear that many of them then had no idea that any effective medical treatment existed.

So I began to accept that I must write a book – but not as an act of exorcism. HRT may have haunted, pursued and possessed me, but it was no pale ghost to be laid by the power of the word.

On the contrary, the book had to show Hormone Replacement Therapy as a firm reality, a practical working treatment, already changing the lives of countless women. So *No Change* was designed to communicate this reality, to provide shape, form and detail and, above all, to be constructive. It set out to present the facts – to look at the female menopause and at the therapy which could make it obsolete. It weighed the advantages and disadvantages, analysed the support and the opposition. And where possible it tried to do this in human terms, using case-histories interviews and letters. Finally it sought to examine the implications and the future of this biological revolution, both for women and for society.

Although by its very nature *No Change* had to be

written with women in view, it also had men in mind. For the truth is that it is not just women who suffer from the female menopause. Husbands and families suffer as well.

Again it was written for the *lay* reader, but also and hopefully with doctors in mind. For this reason full medical references are given at the back to enable doctors, if they wish, to consult the original papers.

But things move fast in our world today and nowhere more so than in science and medicine. So this new edition has been updated, as any future editions must always be, to include new work and new developments in the HRT field. One major change since publication of the very first edition of *No Change* in June 1975 has been the gradual transfer of HRT prescribing from special menopause clinics into general practice. The conversion of family doctors to the concept of HRT and menopause management has been achieved both through the influence locally of enthusiastic gynaecologists, and nationally via publication in the medical literature of reassuring research and monitoring.

The proliferation of special HRT symposia and postgraduate courses, arranged for GPs across the country, has also played a significant part. Being invited to speak at such meetings provided me with welcome reassurance of the acceptance of *No Change* by the medical profession, but more importantly it allowed me also to hear world experts in the field and be kept abreast of current research and thinking.

It will be obvious by now that *No Change* could never have been an uncommitted book. Eight months after beginning my research in 1972, after visiting medical centres, talking to gynaecologists, endocrinologists and to hundreds of women, some of whom had been on oestrogen replacement for twenty years, I decided the weight of evidence justified my going on HRT myself. If I were to write about it, above all if I were to advocate it, as began to seem likely, I must be prepared to use it myself.

I was, of course, the right age. At fifty-one, I had already experienced two years of very odd symptoms. In my case, hot flushes were mild, but I was afflicted with riveting pains in bones, joints and head, particularly when just dropping off to sleep. These were so severe that they jerked me even out of deep pill-induced sleep. Growing insomnia, depression and a deflating lack of confidence and decision completed a pattern entirely alien to my previous buoyant and rather positive nature. There were times when I really thought I was suffering from some frightful obscure disease, and throughout, though my young doctor was sympathetic, the word menopause was never mentioned and only mild tranquillizers and sleeping pills were prescribed.

Ironically, by the time I knew enough about HRT to be prepared to use it, the worst of this phase of early glandular disturbance and imbalance had passed. But tests revealed I was extremely low in oestrogen and, alert by then to the long-term effects, I went onto HRT more or less as an insurance against future risk of osteoporosis, and in the hope of slowing down other ageing processes.

Since that rather tentative decision back in 1972, my position has become firmer. Not only have I thrived on the treatment personally, but more and more evidence has continued to come in, not just concerned with the short-term effect of Hormone Replacement in eliminating the common menopausal symptoms we are familiar with, but concerned with the long-term protection I was looking for against the deep-seated and unseen changes, known to be associated with oestrogen deficiency. And evidence has increased to indicate the protective role of oestrogen against some of the serious diseases, to which women become more vulnerable after the menopause.

My confidence has been boosted still further, by finding that not only in America, but in Britain as well, top men, men like Sir John Peel, the Queen's former gynaecologist, had been quietly using this therapy for their patients for many years.

So while *No Change* has endeavoured to present all the medical, social and economic arguments both for and against HRT, to enable readers to make up their own minds, my own position is clear.

It is quite simple. I believe there is a special charge on doctors and on modern medicine to bring effective help to women in relation to the menopause and the years that follow. It is, after all, modern medicine which has created the present situation, in which women in the developed world now live, on average, to around seventy-eight years. That can mean a third of a lifetime deprived of oestrogen. It is the duty of modern medicine to ensure that the extra years it has won for them are lived comfortably and fully, not crippled and limited by the effects of oestrogen deficiency.

I believe that women have the right to age in a way that parallels the ageing process of a man, with no abrupt decline, no accelerated ageing, and no atrophy of the sex organs to make intercourse painful, sexual response impossible, and middle-aged marriage a misery.

But the task of the book is really to set out the choice. The fact that women have such a choice, at last, is enough to make someone burst into print as well as into praise.

What can't be cured must be endured, and in the past women did just that. Now for the first time in history, where the menopause is concerned, they do not have to. They can decide for themselves whether their menopause is really necessary. Some will still feel it is. They will reject on principle a routine which involves them in a daily pill, a twice weekly patch, or a six monthly implant. Others, with only mild menopause symptoms, will also prefer to let nature take its course.

But there will be many who are suffering severely, and others who are simply motivated towards staying as young as possible as long as possible, who will feel that Hormone Replacement is for them. Still others will just derive benefit from the fact that a choice exists, from the knowledge that if things become too bad effective help can be given. The existence of the choice in itself springs the trap, reduces tension.

Many women readers will already be familiar with HRT in concept if not in practice. So for them this book will reinforce existing knowledge about both the menopause and its treatment; in addition it will provide details of the latest research findings and of the wide range of new HRT products available.

For those women, who have either not heard of HRT or only read superficial and sometimes sensational reports, I hope *No Change* will help to redress the balance. It will explain how HRT works, which oestrogens are suitable and the difference between these and the more powerful kind needed for the contraceptive pill. It will explain variations in methods of administration and the ways in which oestrogen can be combined with other hormones, such as progesterone, to provide essential safeguards and testosterone to improve libido, where this is required.

Finally for every woman, I hope this book will make clear that she no longer, unless she chooses, need be fobbed off during the menopause with prescriptions for palliatives such as aspirin, Librium or Valium, or worse still dismissed with the words, 'It's just your age. There is nothing to be done. You must put up with it.'

There is a great deal to be done. You don't have to put up with it. The choice is *yours*.

Chapter 1

Biological lib

Freud said, 'Biology is destiny'. No woman is going to argue with that. They are all too familiar with the truth of it in their own experience. From puberty, onwards, women are constantly, in one way or another, the victims and the prisoners of their own biology.

But it is equally true in terms of the evolution of the human race. The fact that men, as young adults, proved to be bigger, taller and stronger than women, not unnaturally enabled them to assume the dominant role. By contrast, female biology, the lighter physique, but above all the crippling limitations imposed by reproductive functions, prevented women from successfully challenging the existing situation – until now.

In the past the long, dangerous and weakening years of repeated child-bearing and caring kept women first from the hunting pack, and later from the councils of power. And it has gone on much the same way ever since, despite the female conceit (or is it crafty male deceit?) that 'the hand that rocks the cradle rules the world'. Except for a few exceptional women, most female hands have been too tired or too empty of gold to shape their own lives, let alone shape history. No wonder they have fallen back, all too literally, on the precarious politics of the bedroom, exerting oblique influence on men and events as and when they could.

And then in this century, tentatively at first and always in the face of opposition, women began to be given the chance to control the biology which had for so long controlled them. The first glimmerings of Biological Lib came with the better hygiene, better medical care and the development of anaesthetics, which gradually reduced the danger and the pain of childbirth. It was Queen Victoria, too often and unjustly remembered only as a symbol of prudery, who gave anaesthesia respectability and impetus, by having chloroform administered for a royal birth, and so helped to defeat the sanctimonious 'against nature' lobby.

It was this same 'against nature' argument which in this century was raised again, first to oppose contraception and later to obstruct Hormone Replacement.

The battle for modern contraception has been won, and the old hit-and-miss methods have given way to the highly efficient and widely used intra-uterine device and the contraceptive pill. These techniques do not rely on suspect barriers, but enable women to manipulate and control their own biology. The IUD prevents any fertilized egg implanting itself in the wall of the uterus, and the contraceptive pill ingeniously raises the female hormone levels to stimulate those of pregnancy, so that ovulation is prevented just as it would be in a real pregnancy.

So women in their fertile years have achieved for the first time the ability to control their own biology, to plan their families and their lives, and compete at last on something like equal terms with men.

But evolution has set another brake on female enterprise and energy, coming into operation in mid-life in the form of the menopause. More correctly, the whole process of degeneration, starting with the atrophy and shut-down of the ovaries and continuing through to old age, is known as the climacteric. The menopause strictly means only 'final menstruation', but because it is accepted among women and in common parlance to have the wider meaning, the term is used in that sense also throughout this book.

So, with Biological Lib within the grasp of the younger woman who wants it, the same knowledge of the complex chemistry and workings of the sex hormones, which led to the development of the contraceptive pill, has now been used to bring about a second biological revolution, just as radical and profound for the older woman.

Most revolutions are designed to bring about change, this one is designed to prevent 'the change of life'. Again, the concept is beautifully and ingeniously simple, and again it relies on artificially manipulating the female hormone levels.

It was known that the menopause came about as the result of the decline in the number of stored ova or eggs. Every girl baby is born complete with her generous endowment of potential ova, numbering several hundred thousand. But of these only some four hundred actually mature and once they are used up, that is that. Fertility is over. The ovaries respond to new instructions and begin to close down, so that the production of the two vital female sex hormones, oestrogen and progesterone, declines. The result is an irregular menstrual pattern and finally an end to the monthly cycle.

Unfortunately, it is also the beginning of glandular imbalance and the familiar menopause symptoms. It is the beginning too of more deep-seated changes in the body which take place in the post-menopause years, and which come about due to lack of circulating oestrogen.

After the menopause, the ovaries become small and shrivelled, the lining of the womb atrophic and the vaginal skin thin and more vulnerable to infection. The vagina itself narrows and the external skin also becomes thin and less sexually responsive. The mucous membrane of the bladder also takes part in this pelvic atrophy, and the resulting thinning of the sensitive bladder neck contributes to urinary frequency and urgency which sometimes occurs in older women.

The degenerative changes in the skin also show elsewhere, the loss of subcutaneous fat gives rise to extensive wrinkling, with the skin becoming dry, scaly and inelastic. Absence of oestrogen, also causes breasts to become flabby, while the nipples flatten out and become non-erectile. It also permits a rise in bone resorption leading to thin and brittle bones (osteoporosis) in later years.

Until scientists succeed in tampering with the biological clock, a still distant prospect, the shut-down of the ovaries cannot be prevented. Meanwhile, though restoring oestrogen could not restore fertility (and few women in mid-life would want that) it could restore normal pre-menopause oestrogen levels. If the wretched symptoms so many women experienced were really due to oestrogen deficiency, then restoring it should eliminate them. It did. In practice the concept was found to work exactly as gynaecologists who pioneered it had predicted. Hot flushes were eliminated, vaginal atrophy relieved, and increased resorption of bone prevented. In fact the body was restored to premenopausal hormone balance and pre-menopausal harmony.

But it was one thing to prove that it worked, and quite another to get a traditionally minded medical profession to accept the revolutionary idea of the menopause as a deficiency condition that needed treating. After all, over the centuries the 'change' had been considered as a natural and inevitable part of ageing, a normal state for a woman at a certain time of life. No one ever bothered to consider the cause, in fact, age itself was considered cause enough, until modern endocrinology and a new understanding of hormones suggested otherwise.

The man in the forefront of the biological revolution to make the menopause obsolete, expounding the concept, putting it into practice and fighting to gain for it both acceptance and respectability, was a British-born gynaecologist, Robert Wilson, working in New York. As Consultant in Obstetrics and Gynaecology at four big New York hospitals, he began his first investigation half a century ago.

He believed rightly that the menopause had been largely neglected by medicine because some women never develop serious problems; those who do, and even dare to complain, are too often treated by doctors as hypochondriacs. There was some justification for the traditional view of the menopause as an unavoidable part of ageing, when nothing effective could be done to help. But Dr Wilson felt that the new discoveries should be changing these *laissez-faire* medical attitudes. He set out quite deliberately to shock what he called the 'nice-Nellies' of either sex, many of them doctors, by describing the menopausal women as 'castrates' deprived of sexual function. And he went on to draw a horrifying picture of the post-menopausal woman, liable to drying tissues, weakening muscles, sagging skin, brittle bones and shrinking vagina.

If there was an element of over-statement in all this, at least as shock tactics it worked. And by administering oestrogens, first by injection and later orally, he proved that many of the changes believed to be an integral part of middle age in women, could be prevented and even reversed. In fact part of his credo, imparted with almost messianic zeal, was that Hormone Replacement Therapy ideally should be seen as preventative medicine, to forestall the onset of the menopause before it even happened.

During the 1950s and 1960s, Dr Wilson not only put his concept widely into practice, but kept up a flow of medical papers and articles on the subject, and finally set up the Wilson Foundation, a non-profit making organization, dedicated to funding and inspiring both research and propaganda concerned with HRT. It was a stirring and successful crusade, and it culminated in 1966 with him becoming author of a best-seller called *Feminine Forever*, published in Britain by W. H. Allen and in America by M. Evans.

Dr Wilson's book was based strongly not only on

his convictions and attitudes as a doctor, but on his convictions and attitudes as a man, betraying a romantic regard that amounts almost to reverence for that mysterious core of womanhood which he calls 'femininity'. This quality, a subtle blend of the sexual and emotional rooted deep in our correct hormone balance, could be, he believes, cruelly extinguished by what he terms the 'castrating' effects of the menopause, leaving a neutered and devalued creature, deserving man's pity rather than his passion.

Writing as a woman for other women, and also writing almost ten years later in the age of Women's Liberation, my own approach was inevitably less romantic and more rational, with perhaps less emphasis on femininity and more on feminism, and the right of women to more say in decisions medical or social which affect their own bodies and their own lives.

Also, nothing as dynamic as Hormone Replacement Therapy, subject to wide use and wide research, can ever stand still, and some of the thinking and some of the details of technique have changed since Robert Wilson first launched his campaign and wrote his major papers. But his basic concept is still triumphantly vindicated by results, and when I met him in New York in March of 1972, I met a man whose battle was well on the way to being won on the American continent.

However, though he was then approaching seventy-five, he made it clear he would go on campaigning until full acceptance for HRT was achieved throughout the world, and most especially in his country of birth, Great Britain. He estimated then that it might be another ten years before the majority of the British medical profession were converted to the concept.

Although the majority of gynaecologists in the US at that time were convinced advocates of HRT, there were also some who had reservations about long-term use and would only prescribe for short periods. At family doctor level, particularly in country areas, there was still resistance based on either apathy or ignorance.

Despite this, the United States led the world in use of Hormone Replacement at the menopause, with Canada, South Africa and West Germany not far behind. After them came Italy, France, Brazil, Mexico and Japan, while Great Britain, incredibly for such a medically advanced country, was still somewhere at the bottom of the league, below even the Philippines.

Today Britain leads the world in HRT know-how, though not yet in prescribing levels. Dr Wilson's estimate of ten years to convert GPs proved to be optimistic. In that time only the top British specialists were won over, and it was to take another ten years before the majority of GPs were to become convinced of the safety of HRT as well as of its effectiveness.

Taking part with me in the popular BBC radio programme *You and Yours*, Dr Gerald Swyer, a leading British endocrinologist, and then consultant at University College Hospital, London stated:

There are many women who from the menopause onwards experience significant deficiency in oestrogen. There is no question whatever that for them Hormone Replacement Therapy is the specially indicated treatment. Apart from relieving immediate symptoms, we have good reason to believe that much of the osteoporosis (brittling of bones) experienced by older women can be relieved by oestrogen replacement, and there is also a prophylactic effect against cardio-vascular disease.

The words of great men carry great weight and are powerful weapons in any war. This book will be quoting from many such authorities. But the part women themselves have played and must continue to play must never be underestimated. In the 1970s it was pressure from British women, once they knew HRT could relieve miserable menopause symptoms, that overwhelmed GP surgeries and finally forced the first British menopause clinics into existence. With them came the vital research that was to set safe prescribing guidelines.

In the 1990s, with acceptance by doctors of the long-term protection HRT affords to bones and heart, women could help once more by adding their support to the concept of oestrogen replacement as part of preventive medicine, used early enough and long enough to short-circuit the onset of conditions that can too often prematurely cripple and kill.

To have the confidence to do this and reap the long-term benefits, it helps to understand the basic and benign role of oestrogen in a woman's life. It is the hormone that holds the key to a woman's health and happiness, and it is at work in the body even before birth.

Chapter 2

The role of oestrogen – the making of a woman

It is no exaggeration to say that the powerful female sex hormone, oestrogen, is crucial in forming and maintaining a woman, and it begins its work as early as six months before birth, to influence the growing foetus in the female direction.

Although oestrogen is totally essential to complete this differentiation, gender and sex are actually determined at the very moment of conception along with all other characteristics.

The marvellous mechanism of heredity is so interrelated with the action of oestrogen, and the two stories are so fascinating, compelling and interwoven, that I shall make no apology for combining them here.

When you consider the billions of people alive today, the great procession that has gone before and the vast numbers that will come after, it is not easy to accept the fact that there is no one in the world quite like you, never has been and never will be again. You are unique. And if you think that is a line in smooth flattery, you are wrong. It is the simple truth; a hard statement of scientific fact, rooted in the laws of genetics and mathematics.

The process is a curious mixture of the random and the precise. Nothing in the biological sense could be more random than the coming together of the two people who are to be the parents. Yet this one man and this one woman are each unique, carrying their own special blueprints, precisely written and coded on pairs of genes, which are strung like beads on the twenty-three pairs of chromosomes contained in each cell in the body.

There is just one special type of cell, the mature sex cells (the ova in the female and the sperm in the male) which are different. In those there are only twenty-three *single* chromosomes bearing *single* genes, so that when a sperm fertilizes an egg and the genetic packages from each parent come together, the fusion results again in twenty-three *pairs* of chromosomes. The genes also pair off once more, but in a new alignment to form an entirely new blueprint for a new and different person.

As the foetus is formed, these genes control factors like hair colour, hair type, eye colour, eye shape, nose shape, blood type, height and, indeed, every single characteristic.

It would be impossible (and far too complicated), even to try to follow the chain-gangs of worker genes as they direct, organize and specialize from the one original cell to the twenty-six trillion cells which go to make up a newborn baby. But each time the cells divide to form new ones, into them go exact replicas of all the chromosomes and all the genes. Many have work to do in every cell, but others only go into action if they are in a cell where their special craft is needed, making pigment for instance or perhaps forming bone or transmitting messages.

But one set of instructions is absolutely fundamental and this must be followed, because it is the one that determines sex and so for a woman initiates the oestrogen story.

Among the twenty-three pairs of chromosomes carried in every cell, there is one special pair of sex chromosomes. In women these are both of one type called X, and so the pair together form an XX combination. In men, however there are two kinds, the familiar X type and a smaller Y type, giving an XY chromosome pair.

In the egg and the sperm, as we have seen, the

pairs of chromosomes are split up. In the egg the sex chromosome must always be an X type, because this is the only sort a woman possesses. But among male sperm, some carry X type and some Y type in equal proportions.

So it is easy to see that it is the father, by the chance donation of either an X or Y sperm, who determines the sex of the baby. If a Y sperm wins the procreation race to penetrate and fertilize the female egg, which already contains its own X chromosome, this XY pair of chromosomes will produce a boy. If an X-bearing sperm is the first to reach the egg, the XX constitution makes a girl.

Despite this, to begin with and for some three months after conception, everyone is actually bisexual, equipped with the rudimentary organs and ducts for both sexes and capable of development in either direction. Only during the fourth month of life in the womb does nature's computer switch the foetus along a single-sex road. Programmed by an XY chromosome, it commands the male organs and ducts to develop, leaving the female counterparts in their rudimentary state. Programmed by an XX chromosome, it triggers development of the female organs, leaving the male structure untouched. But once this sexual differentiation is begun, the sex hormones secreted by the growing testes or ovaries take over, and continue to govern the direction of development both before birth, and again later during puberty.

It is interesting that adults still retain some reminders of these bisexual beginnings. A man has clearly formed but non-functioning nipples, and a woman the clitoris, which is really the undeveloped penis.

One of the most fascinating bits of information, which modern knowledge has revealed and which must delight feminists, is that, quite contrary to biblical mythology, it is the female which is the basic sex. It is now known that left to itself every foetus would turn towards the female. Only the powerful and continuous intervention of the male sex hormones, the androgens, effect the differentiation which results in a boy. So the legend of Lilith is after all more appropriate than that of Adam.

A male gynaecologist commenting on this, pointed out that rather less delightfully for Women's Lib, the female can be regarded as the neuter sex and the male as the positive and more advanced differentiation!

Whichever way you care to look at it, although the prototype female is already the basic sex, oestrogen must be present and in the right quantities, to ensure this female foetus developing fully and correctly.

In fact, the balance between male and female hormones is crucial, both before birth and throughout life, and this fact too is related to continuing bisexual potential. Everyone produces some hormones of the other sex. Men produce small amounts of oestrogen and women secrete small amounts of androgens. So if at any time there is a failure to produce enough of the right sex hormones to maintain the balance in the proper direction, there can be a tilt towards the opposite sex.

The foetus is particularly vulnerable in this respect. Too much oestrogen reaching a male foetus can result in feminization, and equally, too much androgen reaching the female foetus can mean a girl baby being born with masculine traits, maybe even an enlarged clitoris, which in the past could sometimes tragically lead to wrong assignment of sex.

Fortunately, such sexual ambiguity is rare, but the fact that it can occur and the reasons for it, do serve to emphasize the power and importance of the sex hormones.

The fate of the male castrate throughout history offers another striking illustration. Deprived, either deliberately or through accident, of his normal supply of male hormones before puberty, the boy always retains a high voice, develops female-pattern body hair and has no beard growth.

Hormonal imbalance sometimes shows up clearly for the first time at puberty, with a girl failing to show the usual budding breasts or menstruation; or with a boy failing to develop facial hair and deepening voice. Fortunately today, modern endocrine knowledge provides the answer to such lack of development or to late maturation. Appropriate hormone treatment is given, and maintained if necessary to correct the situation.

The menopause on occasions offers a similar example of hormone imbalance at work. In some older women declining oestrogen levels can tilt the balance so far towards the male that the growth of facial hair is triggered and occasionally the voice too is affected, becoming low and gruff. A very charming woman, whom I know well, found her voice affected in this way after the menopause. She told me, 'It led to ridiculous confusion on the telephone. I was always being mistaken for my husband or my son. I tried to keep a sense of humour, but it was pretty shattering to be called Mr.'

Hormone Replacement Therapy quickly corrected the voice problem for her. It can often also help with facial hair. But it is simpler, if possible, to *prevent* the imbalance and hirsuteness. Once the hair follicles have been triggered, it is not always easy to stop the growth.

All this could seem to present a daunting picture, but it should be remembered that, for most people, nature's computer works well and the direction of sexual development and drive is clear-cut and normal.

For a girl, oestrogen continues to play a vital role. At first the young ovaries only produce very minute quantities, but such small traces can still be clearly detected in the urine, and it is believed that even these low levels of oestrogen may account for the more rapid skeletal maturation and the earlier onset of puberty, in girls, as opposed to boys.

It is around the age of eleven or twelve, sometimes a little earlier, that the master gland, the pituitary, signals the ovaries to step up oestrogen production.

Just as it once influenced the foetus towards the female, so now the increased oestrogen begins to resculpture the girl into the woman. The flat-chested tomboy is transformed, as breasts and nipples develop, the pelvis widens and fat appears on the hips to give rounded adult contours.

These higher levels of circulating oestrogen also stimulate the growth of external and internal genitalia, secretion of vaginal mucus, pigmentation of the nipples and development of pubic and axillary hair.

But the final act in the drama, the truly sensational transformation scene, comes with the release of the first egg and the establishment of regular menstruation and ovulation. This cyclic monthly rhythm, which becomes so much part of female life, is controlled by a hormonal ebb and flow, involving a complex feedback mechanism between the pituitary and the ovaries.

First the pituitary gland secretes minute quantities of another hormone, known as FSH (follicle-stimulating hormone), a name which describes exactly what it does. Less than a millionth of an ounce a day is sufficient to awaken a few dormant egg cells, and set off a dazzling chain of events.

Around each awakened egg there forms a fluid-filled follicle (a tiny protective sac). Usually only one follicle grows and expands sufficiently to push its way through and actually appear on the surface of the ovary, as a sort of bubble. Where, on rare occasions, two follicles do succeed in doing this, the potential situation exists for conception of non-identical twins.

The growing follicle now secrets more oestrogen to add to that already at work, instructing the uterus (womb) to prepare a thick lining, where any fertilized egg may become implanted and nourished.

The rising levels of oestrogen are sensed by the pituitary and another command goes out. This time yet another hormone, LH (luteinizing hormone), joins FSH and, about mid-cycle, their combined efforts cause the follicle to rupture, releasing the egg, which is swept down through the Fallopian tubes into the uterus.

When the egg breaks out of its follicle it makes quite a tear in the membrane covering the ovary, and some women can actually feel this happen and experience a short sharp pain. When this ovulation occurs there is also a slight rise in temperature. This can be detected and used by women, both in trying to achieve conception or in trying to avoid it, as obviously it signals the time when there is the best chance of bringing the sperm and egg together.

But meanwhile a remarkable process is going on. The scar tissue on the ovary turns into a yellow gland, called the corpus luteum, and this sets about producing that other important female hormone progesterone. Again, the name indicates its main function, for it means pro-gestation or pro-pregnancy, and progesterone is known as the pregnancy hormone. Its main job is to preserve and modify the uterine lining ready for the fertilized egg.

However, if no conception takes place, after about twelve to fourteen days, the corpus luteum dies and the supply of progesterone is shut off, while the level of oestrogen also drops. These changes tell the waiting uterus that no baby has been conceived this time, and so the lining that has been built up is allowed to flow away, and with it the unfertilized egg. This is menstruation.

Needless to say, a mechanism so strong, sturdy and persistent that, against all odds, it has ensured the survival of the human race through a million hostile years, does not give up or become easily discouraged. The hormonal chain of command simply resumes operation – other follicles form – oestrogen levels are raised and the whole process begins again.

From all this, the central role of oestrogen in the life of women is clear, but it goes far beyond this direct control of reproduction. Oestrogen is also carried in the bloodstream to affect every cell in the body.

Protein, the basic substance of all cells, contains nitrogen as one of its most important ingredients, and oestrogen has the invaluable ability of enabling cells to assimilate nitrogen from food more effectively and utilize it more efficiently.

The importance of oestrogen in maintaining what is termed a 'positive nitrogen balance' is recognized in medicine. Oestrogen is administered on occasions to quite young girls, even at the risk of temporary premature maturation, and equally to quite old ladies, to help build up the nitrogen balance and ensure better cell nutrition in certain illnesses.

So the very presence of oestrogen in our bodies helps to ensure healthy cells, and this means, in particular, strong bones and tissues, giving good muscle tone, firm breasts, supple joints, clear skin and shining hair. Perhaps the clearest example of the special bloom oestrogen can give is seen in many women during healthy pregnancies, when oestrogen levels are at their highest.

Some strange and unexpected minor effects of oestrogen were discovered some years ago through the work of a well-known, British zoologist, Professor John Ebling. He has shown that normal women are far more sensitive to the scent of musk, the smell derived from male animals such as the civet, than men are. As this is the basis of most classical perfumes, the sexy scents women use to turn men on probably work indirectly by turning on the women themselves first. The smell had to be a thousand times stronger for a man to notice it than a woman. But if a woman has her ovaries removed, then the scent of musk becomes as faint for her as for a man. Given Hormone Replacement, however, the scent once again becomes vivid and exciting.

Although many of the effects of oestrogen appear to be similarly concerned with keeping women sexually attractive and sexually responsive (both states clearly favoured by evolutionary forces during the fertile years), it does also carry out even more vital tasks, not so readily apparent.

There is, for example, the very specific job which oestrogen, and only oestrogen, can do in maturing the cells of the vagina, keeping it supple, elastic, free from infection and ready for both intercourse and childbirth. Its positive effect in maintaining muscle tone also protects against prolapse and against bladder and urinary problems.

In much the same way, oestrogen is now known to protect our bones against osteoporosis and the heart and arteries against cardio-vascular disease. It has been proved that HRT by restoring oestrogen also restores this protection, reducing bone loss and cutting strokes and heart attacks by 50 per cent.

But the effects of the sex hormones can go beyond the entirely physical into the psychological. Because of the feedback mechanism and the strong link with the pituitary gland, oestrogen and progesterone levels affect emotional stability. It is no coincidence that many women feel depressed, nervy, and irritable just before menstruation, when hormone levels drop. The same kind of reaction can occur at the menopause, and again it is no coincidence that both then and just before menstruation, women have more accidents and commit more crimes. Both this 'pre-menstrual tension', as it is called, and the menopause, respond to hormone treatment.

In many ways oestrogen has a place in the life of a woman rather like that of love itself. When she has them she takes them for granted, realizing their full value only when they are gone.

One eminent British gynaecologist, who was strongly opposed to Hormone Replacement Therapy, told me, 'What a woman needs at the menopause is not oestrogen but a good husband.' It is obviously even better to have both. But while love and husbands cannot be had on prescription or be easily replaced, fortunately, today, oestrogen can.

Chapter 3

Oestrogen deficiency – the long and the short of it

For most women the first sign of the onset of the menopause, usually occurring in their mid- to late forties, is a change in the pattern of menstruation. If this has been regular, it becomes less so; if it has been irregular, it becomes more so; for other women the periods may just come at increasingly longer intervals, be unusually heavy, or simply become scanty and perhaps dark in colour, until eventually, they cease altogether. The whole process may last for as long as five years, though in a few cases menstruation just ceases abruptly with no prior warning.

This abrupt cessation happens, of course, in the case also of women who undergo an operation involving removal of ovaries or where ovaries are destroyed by irradiation. Both a surgical menopause or radium menopause bring a rapid fall in oestrogen levels, and often the swift onset of symptoms.

Not all women suffer all symptoms, and this is really just as well, for there are some twenty-one recognized symptoms associated with the menopause. There are even some women who seem to sail through the change of life with no problems at all. These are the fortunate ones, estimated at around 15 per cent, whose adrenal glands seem able to step up production of oestrogen precursors, sufficiently to compensate for failing ovaries. These are converted to oestrogen in fatty tissue, so for once plump women are on the winning side. Eventually, however, though at a much later stage, oestrogen deficiency usually catches up with them too, though it may not by then produce any overt symptoms.

For the rest, the other 85 per cent, symptoms most common at the onset of the menopause are fatigue, headaches, irritability, palpitations, dizziness and, to a lesser degree, depression. These mark the beginning of the disturbances arising from hormone imbalance.

Hot flushes (or flashes, which somehow sounds more dramatic) night sweats, and pains in the joints and muscles usually come rather later, in the early post-menopause, that is soon after ovarian function and menstruation have ceased.

Another very strange symptom which many women have mentioned to me is officially called 'formication' – a word which demands rather careful spelling! It is the medical term for the peculiar crawling sensation near the body surface, which one American woman described to me as feeling like 'an army of ants walking about under your skin'.

An interesting piece of research, the first of its kind, but still relevant, was carried out some time ago by the International Health Foundation, to study the attitude of women towards the menopause in five European countries – a sort of menopausal Common Market. The study was based on personal interviews with two thousand women, all between the ages of forty-six and fifty-five, from Belgium, France, Great Britain, Italy and West Germany.

Questions were asked about memories of their mothers' experiences, about their own experiences, and about their attitudes towards the menopause and life after it. They were also asked how much they knew about medical treatment available, and if they had sought such help.

Some fascinating culture differences emerged, with British women, in proverbial stiff upper lip tradition, taking the most optimistic and stoical view. The women of Belgium and Italy were the most gloomy, and in particular, twice as many of them thought the menopause marked not only the start of old age, but the end of their attractiveness to men.

The symptoms most commonly experienced throughout the menopause proved to be: 55 per cent flushes, 43 per cent tiredness, 41 per cent nervousness, 39 per cent sweating, 38 per cent headaches, 32 per cent insomnia, 30 per cent depression, 29 per cent irritability, 25 per cent joint and muscle pains, 24 per cent dizziness, 24 per cent palpitations and 22 per cent pins and needles, which is perhaps similar to the tingling, crawling sensation.

Over all, it is interesting to find that although 86 per cent said they suffered during the menopause, only 52 per cent had actually sought medical help. Obviously intensity and duration of symptoms must partly determine this, but it also seems likely that the numbers seeking help are related to the numbers knowing that such help existed. Only 53 per cent knew there was any medical treatment to lessen the problems of the menopause, and British women were particularly ill-informed. Only 36 per cent of British women had heard of any medical treatment as against 71 per cent in West Germany, 57 per cent in Belgium, 54 per cent in France and 47 per cent in Italy.

Among those who knew treatment existed, the West Germans were the best informed. Sixty-six per cent of those who knew also actually mentioned oestrogen replacement or hormone treatment, while the comparative figures for those who had heard of HRT in the other countries were 41 per cent in Italy, 40 per cent in France, 22 per cent in Belgium and Great Britain. A snap survey done for this book confirmed a similar percentage of women in the USA experiencing menopause symptoms, but a far greater number aware of the possibility of hormonal help. The high profile given to HRT over recent years in this country has considerably raised awareness though not yet sufficiently about long-term benefits.

Earlier this century, in fact up to the second world

war, the average age for final menstruation was around forty-eight. Recent surveys, including one among over 6000 women in Holland, have shown this age has risen now to over fifty-one. With earlier puberty this means the fertile life of women is extending at both ends, perhaps to match the longer life expectancy. The Dutch survey also found that while 23 per cent of women aged forty-one were already starting to experience irregular menstruation, approximately half of the women aged forty-six, forty-seven and forty-eight still reported their menstrual cycles as regular. After that, however, the percentage with regular cycles decreases rapidly.

Although research and surveys reveal a general basic pattern in both onset and symptoms, the menopause experience for each woman remains intensely individual. Not only does severity, duration and number of symptoms vary for everyone, but so does reaction, attitude and situation.

The hot flushes, which one woman may tolerate well within home and family, can be quite intolerable and embarrassing to a woman holding down a job which involves contact with the public or with male colleagues.

Both the International Health Foundation survey and my own enquiries confirm that most women worry as much about the psychological aspects of the change of life as about the physical. It is worrying to be subject to sweating and headaches, to put on weight or lose that once firm figure, but it is just as worrying to lose one's memory, lack confidence or become subject to confusion and depression.

Barbara Simpson, deputy head of a large mixed comprehensive school in England, wrote to me after my series of articles first appeared, and her case not only illustrated this point, but emphasized the difference between the American and the British scene. She wrote,

... I was working in America and was put on Premarin

(natural oestrogen) immediately following my
hysterectomy over there three years ago. I was absolutely
fine, physically and mentally, until I came back to England,
where to my horror my own doctor insisted I come off the
therapy. He gradually cut down the dosage until I was off
it completely. I soon became aware of hot flushes and more
gradually of growing confusion, lack of memory and lack
of confidence. In my job, working with male colleagues and
boys of up to sixteen, the flushes which made me go red
and hot were very embarrassing. But even worse was the
growing inability to concentrate. You can imagine in this
job, I have to keep right on top. Needless to say I have been
back to my doctor but he adamantly refuses to renew the
prescription and I am becoming desperate. Now I know
from your article that the therapy is obtainable in this
country. I am determined to change my doctor . . .

Barbara Simpson was an intelligent and determined
woman and once she knew Hormone Replacement *was*
available she obtained it, and reported back to me that
it worked like a miracle and she was again thriving.
She went privately to a gynaecologist, and later also
changed to another group practice of GPs, where the
doctors, although not too familiar with the treatment,
were at least prepared to carry out the gynaecologist's
recommended regime.

One of the most distressing physical symptoms of
oestrogen deficiency which women experience very
often after surgical removal of ovaries, and also in the
natural post-menopause, is vaginal dryness and atrophy,
often so severe that intercourse becomes painful or
impossible.

It seems possible that the medical profession under-
estimates this problem, because so many letters I
receive mention it and also stress the fact that the
writers are too shy to discuss it with their doctors. I
have suggested in my talks to GPs at Menopause Symposia that where a woman complains of *other*
menopause symptoms, it can sometimes help if they
then follow up by asking her if she experiences any

problem with pain on intercourse. This question raised quite matter-of-factly usually encourages discussion of a subject she may have felt too embarrassed to mention herself.

Because this is one of the symptoms most closely and directly linked to lack of oestrogen, and one which is effectively and swiftly relieved, either by oestrogen tablets taken orally, or by oestrogen cream applied locally, it is particularly tragic that it should so often go untreated. The lubricants and vaginal jellies sometimes prescribed are, at best, only palliatives, and do nothing to remove the basic cause. Oestrogen replacement can relieve the condition within weeks. Replacement Therapy started early enough, of course, prevents it ever happening.

Dozens of women wrote desperate and moving letters about this problem, many of them showing clearly how this menopause symptom in particular casts a long shadow, beyond the woman herself, to darken and endanger both marriage and family stability.

A typical letter from a fifty-year-old English woman ran:

Your articles on Hormone Replacement Therapy brought me the first hope in five years. I began the menopause five years ago. Since then I have suffered not only the usual physical symptoms, particularly back-aches and night sweats, but also insomnia, confusion and depression.

My doctor says it is 'natural' and 'just my age', and gives me pain-killers for my back and Librium for what he calls my 'bad nerves'. All his treatment does is make me more tired, so that I get more irritable.

I love my husband and two sons very much but I know I have become a misery to live with.

I used to enjoy a normal sex life, but now it is something I dread because it is so painful. Recently I bought twin beds, pretending it was because I was so restless, but really it was to avoid him wanting me.

I am truly afraid for my marriage if this goes on, and my doctor refuses even to read your article or consider giving

me oestrogen. I do a part-time job and would be happy to
pay for the treatment if it would help me back to normal.
My family can't understand my misery.

This woman finally received help, and took the trouble
to write to me happily a few months later to say she
had been to a doctor in London who specialized in
Hormone Replacement. After a test to establish that
her oestrogen levels were low, he had put her on natural
oestrogen. Within weeks 'life became worth living
again', to use her own phrase.

Depression is a symptom which many women complain about in their letters. By no means all middle-
aged depression is hormone-based, and this will be
discussed in greater detail in later chapters. But some
of it is essentially rooted in the disturbances which
oestrogen deprivation causes in the autonomic nervous
system. The case of Mrs Joan Williams illustrates this
well. Aged fifty-five when I met her, she had been
struggling since the end of menstruation five years
before with terrible night sweats and palpitations. She
told me,

It was so bad that I could only sleep if I was drugged. All
my doctor would do, and it was a woman doctor, was give
me Librium and Valium to help me sleep. She said she
couldn't do anything else, it was 'just my age'. The worst
part was the awful depression and lack of confidence. I got
that I couldn't go out or talk to anyone, I just wanted to curl
up and sleep the day away . . .
    I did fight against it, I struggled at first to look after my
home and go out to work, because I didn't want to give
in. My husband didn't understand, and all he would say was,
'Pull yourself together'. In the end I just had to give up the
job. I felt so ill and desperate that I really thought I was
going to die.
    Then I read your articles in the *Birmingham Mail*. I'd got
a bit of money saved from my job and my husband said
he'd give anything to get me back to normal, so we decided
I should go privately to a gynaecologist. It wasn't after all

very expensive, but I can't tell you what it was like to have someone to talk to who really understood. You see, I really thought I might be going off my head. In fact I'd even asked my own doctor if I could pay to go and see a psychiatrist. Then that gynaecologist explained it all, and told me other women felt the same way. She gave me a thorough examination, checked my oestrogen level and put me on the Hormone Replacement. Within two weeks the physical symptoms had gone completely. After all these years I could hardly believe it.

Quite soon the depression lifted and then I began to get my confidence back. Now I am planning to start a job again. My husband is amazed to see me taking an interest in my hair again and in my looks. He understands now that it was a physical thing, not just something in my mind.

Thank goodness I don't get that sort of letter so often these days. Just an occasional unhappy letter betrays the fact that a few blinkered, and usually elderly, GPs have not kept up with the medical literature and still retain old misguided fears and prejudices.

The last chapter referred briefly to the protection oestrogen gives against bladder and urinary problems, and striking confirmation of this came in 1988, in a letter from Angela Kilmartin, whose work and books on cystitis have helped so many sufferers from this miserable condition.

It isn't well known that a common, but largely unrecognized symptom or problem of menopause/hysterectomy is cystitis. It can be bacterial or non-bacterial. Both sorts are due to ageing skin. We don't just wrinkle externally as we get older we also 'wrinkle', dry-up and slightly shrink inside as well.

Some specialists like to stretch (dilate) the urethral tube and the bladder – BEWARE! Once started it has to be done more often. No! This is the old way – the best way to help is again through HRT. As the skin regains tone and elasticity in treatment, the urethra and bladder will stop 'twinging' too.

Over the years in my work with women who suffer from

cystitis, about one third of all of them start cystitis in the menopause or following a hysterectomy. Many of these women have had negligent medical care in not receiving assessments or not being allowed a three month experiment on HRT. Those who have had better and enlightened help either from GP or gynaecologist have made substantial or full recovery not only from cystitis but, of course, the other miserable symptoms as well. From the mildest oral tablet treatment through to the full-blown implant, help can be extremely effective.

I always used to wonder how my own body would react to menopausal years, well, now I know! Aged 46 I have started on Prempack .625 mg for depressive feelings, aching knees, tired and dark eyes, crawling tiredness and shaky periods. After my second month pack, my tiredness is abating, I have lost five pounds weight, my knees don't hurt any more, I'm sleeping eight to nine hours a night without disturbance and I'm much brighter.

Push for it, is my advice, even if the blood test for hormone levels seems all right. That's what I did and I've been proved right!

Thank you for your wonderful work on menopause/hysterectomy. I think we women know as much about ourselves these days as 'specialists'.

Best wishes, *Angela Kilmartin*

Talking to Angela again for this later edition, I found she is still busy lecturing and counselling, deservedly recognized by doctors as a 'specialist' in her field. She still enthuses about the benefits of HRT and about the fact that women today no longer have to fight to get this treatment as they once did.

With such a change for the better in medical attitudes and with most GPs now prescribing, no woman need fall victim to the short- or long-term effects of oestrogen deficiency.

So far all the symptoms discussed, both mental and physical, have been the sort which show up clearly and quickly, and of which a woman is only too well aware herself. But there are others, unseen and insidious, which in the long term can cause far more serious problems.

Chapter 4

Long-term protection

Symptoms which can be seen and felt can be dealt with in one way or another. A woman suffering from lack of energy or headaches can find relief either by taking more rest or, if this does not work, seeking help from her doctor. She is aware of what is happening, and the problem is usually controllable.

Far more frightening and disconcerting is the stealthy and secret onset of the condition known as osteoporosis, the medical term for 'porous bones'. This results from accelerated loss of healthy bone after the menopause, with the victim not even aware that it is happening. The first warning that her bones are becoming weak and brittle can be a fracture of the wrist or the hip, after only a light fall, or the onset of spinal osteoporosis heralded by low-back pain. As the vertebrae continue to crumble and crush, there may be a height loss of several inches, and often acute pain.

It was the fact that women who had their ovaries removed developed osteoporosis very early in their lives that first linked the disease to lack of sex hormones. Also, women develop it far more often and far earlier than men, and this was correctly thought to be related to the later and slower decline of male sex hormones, which allowed their parallel protective role to last longer.

Osteoporosis is *ten* times more common in women than in men, and this is reflected in the tenfold rise in Colles fractures of the wrist, recorded for women over fifty, with no similar rise in fractures for men of that age. Women usually have a smaller bone mass than men to start with, of course, but the real damage is done by the menopause.

Even so, not all women become osteoporotic with age, but the proportion that is affected is frighteningly high. One in four develop brittle bones after the age of fifty, and a recent survey by the National Osteoporosis Society reveals the average age of first fractures is as low as sixty. By the age of seventy, one in two women have already suffered some form of osteoporotic fracture, with the rate for broken hips soaring. Hip fractures are very common in women, because the narrow neck of the femur (hip bone) is extremely vulnerable, with age becoming so demineralized and porous that it suddenly snaps. And it doesn't necessarily take a fall for this to happen. The femur can simply and quite spontaneously fracture as body weight is transferred briefly from one foot to another in the process of walking.

The incidence of female hip fractures in recent years has been around 35,000 annually; but rates are rising rapidly, and the number of women estimated to fall victim annually in the 1990s is over 50,000. Of these, *20 per cent* will die, and of those who survive, *50 per cent* will never again be able to lead independent lives.

This sort of pain, deformity and premature death inflicted on women by osteoporosis would be tragic in any circumstances, but the fact that post-menopausal osteoporosis is *100 per cent preventable* makes the present situation both tragic and intolerable. I was delighted to see a lead being given, as it so often is, by our splendid Women's Institute, who passed a strong resolution at one of their national annual general meetings, calling for better prevention and treatment of osteoporosis, with special emphasis on the wider availability of HRT.

Gynaecologists and GPs today have it within their power virtually to wipe out post-menopausal osteoporosis. Restoring the missing oestrogen restores the protection the bones enjoyed *before* the menopause, and brings bone loss back to pre-menopause levels. In this way, HRT can halt osteoporosis in its tracks.

The medical world is well aware of the vital role oestrogen plays in bone metabolism, interacting with other hormones to help maintain the balance between the two opposing processes that go on throughout life – bone formation and bone resorption.

Once oestrogen is lost, this protective control is lost, and the mineral content of bone, in the form of calcium and phosphate, is leached out at an average rate of two to three per cent a year. In some women, who are fast bone-losers, the rate can even be as high as five per cent a year. So, ten years after ovaries fail, the average woman will have lost 30 per cent of her bone density, and the unlucky fast bone-losers as much as 50 per cent. A lot then depends on the bone mass they started out with, but some 50 per cent will be fast approaching what is termed the 'fracture threshold'.

Apart from fast bone-losers, the women most at risk of developing clinical osteoporosis are those who suffer an early natural or surgical menopause. This is because of the extra years during which accelerated bone loss is able to take place. For these women, HRT is mandatory. It has been shown that women who run into a premature menopause, and have failed to take HRT, carry four times the normal risk of brittle bones and repeated fractures.

As mentioned earlier, in addition to the cost in terms of suffering to women, there is the cost to the NHS of coping with the consequences of osteoporosis. This has risen from an estimated £500 million a year in the 1980s to over £800 million a year in the mid-1990s.

Statistics show that the incidence of osteoporosis is increasing in *both* sexes, and at a rate not entirely accounted for by our ageing population. Clearly, other factors are at work, almost certainly the more sedentary lifestyle that many of us lead today, plus a reduction in calcium intake which has followed the switch from dairy to soya or other low fat products. With soaring costs, and NHS facilities in some areas overwhelmed by the numbers of female hip fractures presented for treatment, the Royal College of Physicians recently issued a special report identifying and expressing great concern about what they term 'the osteoporosis epidemic'. *This report not only identified HRT as the only effective way of preventing brittle bones in post-menopausal women, but urged GPs to prescribe it far more widely to control the present crisis.*

As well as reducing suffering, greater use of HRT (which can cost as little as £48 a year) could reduce the financial burden on the NHS and, by cutting hip fracture rates, also free desperately needed beds in female wards, enabling them to be used for other urgent orthopaedic surgery.

Of course, the problem should have been recognized, and HRT brought to the rescue long ago. Even in 1972, when I was researching for the very first edition of this book, plenty of evidence existed that oestrogen could halt this accelerated bone loss in women.

In America, I found a great deal of work had been done on this, particularly by Dr Gilbert Gordan in San Francisco, Professor of Medicine, and Head of both the Endocrine and Bone Clinics, located at the University of California Medical Center.[1] This man is a world expert on osteoporosis, and one of many doctors using HRT successfully both to prevent the onset of osteoporosis, and to combat the established disease.

Dr Gordan told me, 'We find it is the single most effective treatment. We use natural oestrogen, of course, and in the large numbers of women we have treated over many years, a fracture has never been seen once the therapy has been properly instituted and maintained.'

Dr Gordan emphasized that while oestrogen given *early* after the menopause can *prevent* dangerous bone loss and osteoporotic fractures, given *belatedly*, it can only arrest but not reverse the condition. 'Bone once lost cannot be replaced,' he insisted, 'but oestrogen still seems to help reduce the pain and the risk of further fractures.'

There are plenty of examples illustrating the fact that it is never too late. Polly Cartland, the remarkable ninety-seven-year-old mother of British romantic novelist Barbara Cartland (an enthusiastic long-time user and publicist for HRT) was put on oestrogen after breaking a hip in her ninety-sixth year. Barbara Cartland told me, 'I went on oestrogen myself after I had a hysterectomy and felt just wonderful on it. My daughter went on it in her mid-forties as preventative medicine, and my mother was put on it by her doctor to protect against risk of further fractures. So that was three generations of us, all on HRT.'

The redoubtable Barbara herself, when still in her amazingly energetic eighties, quite inadvertently tested HRT's power to protect bone when she suffered a heavy fall without a single bone being broken.

British medicine does at last seem officially to have recognized the role of HRT in preventing post-menopausal bone loss and osteoporosis, but it has taken intensive British medical research behind the scenes, and intensive campaigning up front, through medical seminars and the media, to achieve this. Even now, as we have seen, it still requires the Royal College of Physicians and the Department of Health to prod GPs into wider prescribing of HRT as preventive medicine rather than just to relieve overt symptoms.

Much of the early British work, which confirmed and extended American findings, was carried out at the Mineral Metabolism Unit at Leeds General Infirmary. It was there that Dr Christopher Nordin and Dr John Gallagher set out to determine the actual amount of calcium lost from bone after both natural and surgical menopause (removal of ovaries).

Dr Nordin himself showed me how this was done, by measuring the amounts of calcium excreted in the urine of groups of post-menopausal women, and comparing them with the urine excreted by *pre*-menopausal controls. The tests had to be carried out in the morning, after overnight fasting, to eliminate any of the calcium coming from food. The results, as I could see for myself, showed a dramatic rise in calcium loss in the post-menopausal groups.[2]

Similar results were obtained in Glasgow by Dr J. M. Aitken and his team, this time measuring the actual decrease in bone density using new and accurate scanning devices.[3] Significantly, in both studies, administration of oestrogen was found to bring bone resorption rates rapidly back to pre-menopausal levels.

The Mineral Metabolism Unit at Leeds also went some way towards establishing the mechanism at work. It had already been shown that oestrogen seemed to block resorption of old bone, rather than induce production of new bone. The team at Leeds carried out experiments which demonstrated that one way oestrogen achieves this is by inhibiting the action of another hormone, the parathyroid (PTH), which, unopposed, causes both calcium and phosphate to be leached from bone.

The idea that oestrogen might work to preserve what is called a positive calcium balance, and keep bones healthy, was suggested by the excessive bone loss seen in post-menopausal women with over-active parathyroid glands.[4]

Today it is known that the interaction of oestrogen with other hormones to protect bone is even more complex. As well as blocking the harmful action of parathyroid hormone, it is now recognized that oestrogen also stimulates the liver to produce a protein that reduces the ability of the adrenal hormones to dissolve bone. In addition, it stimulates vitamin D and another hormone, calcitonin, to carry out their special bone-protecting functions.

Until very recently, it was thought, as Dr Gordan had told me, that HRT could *prevent* bone being lost but could not *restore* it. Now, however, there is growing evidence that modern HRT, in what is known as the 'combined' form, which includes progestogen – the oral version of the second female hormone, progesterone – can actively encourage the laying-down of new bone. The basic reason for using 'combined' HRT for any woman with a womb is that the addition of progestogen has been shown to protect the womb lining against the 'over-stimulation', which can occur on oestrogen alone; and this is explained more fully in Chapter 6. Now, several recent reports suggest progestogen used along-side oestrogen seems to encourage formation of new bone,[5] and this could prove another bonus for the com-bined therapy.

In recent years there has been intriguing new evi-dence of another form of HRT showing promise in the battle against osteoporosis. Consultant Gynaecologist, John Studd, and co-workers at King's College Hospital, have just reported an increase in bone density of 8.3 per cent in the spine, and 2.8 per cent in the hip, achieved in just twelve months by treating patients with oestrogen and testosterone (male hormone) implants.[6] The HRT treatment was started early – within two years of the loss of ovarian hormones. Details of this implant technique and of the other advantage testos-terone can confer in increasing libido are detailed later (see Chapter 12).

Today, in the fight against osteoporosis, sophisticated scanners can be used to measure bone density quickly and accurately right at the most vulnerable osteopor-otic sites. Readings taken a few months apart also allow fast bone-losers to be identified. With ninety such machines available by 1995, the DOH special report on osteoporosis urged greater use of these to promote earlier detection and treatment, and also asked for clear guidelines to be set for doctors on prevention and treatment strategies *including* HRT.

Unfortunately, while urging greater use of modern bone scanning techniques, the Department of Health did not offer the extra funding this would require.

Instead the onus was put on fund-holding GP practices and local authorities. It remains to be seen how many will prove willing to underwrite this cost for patients at risk. These would include all who may have undergone premature natural or surgical menopause *without* benefit of HRT, and women who have already suffered a fracture.

Other factors indicating the advisability of a bone scan are a family history of osteoporsis, having small bones rather than large or being thin rather than fat. While such inherited factors have to be accepted as part of life's genetic lottery, it is important they be taken into account when assessing risk status. In the same way doctors must recognize that prolonged use of steroids, often vital to treat asthma or arthritis, has the unwanted side-effect of increasing bone loss.

But there are other adverse factors which you yourself can do something about, such as smoking, heavy drinking, lack of exercise, excess dieting or low calcium intake.

It is particularly important to understand the role of calcium, because although it can never be a substitute for HRT in preventing the accelerated bone loss that follows the menopause (despite suggestions to the contrary in some newspapers) it does have a vital part to play, building and maintaining good bone mass earlier in life, ready to withstand the post-menopausal onslaught.

Unfortunately, in the absence of the female hormones, calcium is not well absorbed, but some studies do suggest that calcium supplements taken *alongside* HRT may confer extra benefit.

This is perhaps the place to pass on a very timely warning issued in 1996 by the British Menopause Society. These doctors, with their special interest and expertise in menopause management, reported increasing worry that some women are being misled by rash marketing claims and press reports advocating so-called 'natural' remedies, vitamin, mineral or herbal, as effective substitutes for HRT. They see particular danger in this for women who have been prescribed replacement therapy specifically for long-term protection to bones or heart, and who are tempted to switch instead to one of the alternative 'remedies'.

Consultant David Sturdee, Chairman of the British Menopause Society, told me, 'Properly controlled trials have confirmed the value of HRT. These other nutritional substances have not undergone formal or rigorous scientific evaluation. There is no scientific evidence to support a change to these therapies. While some of the vitamins and minerals in these products may do women good, on their own they cannot counter the full ravages of oestrogen deficiency, or give the protection against brittle bones and cardio-vascular disease that HRT has been conclusively proven to do.'

Another area of potential danger for any woman with a womb to protect is if they ditch their vital prescribed progestogen in favour of one of the yam-based products, advertised as containing substances similar to this hormone but safer and better. Some of these, neither officially approved nor tested, are being sold through mail order from Ireland to circumvent government medicine control safety regulations. The dosage absorbed is uncertain, effectiveness unproven, and the condition of the womb lining at risk.

These reservations also apply to natural progesterone gel, recently promoted heavily in this country. This product also has undergone no controlled trials or been given a medical licence. Above all, the extraordinary concept that progesterone deficiency rather than oestrogen deficiency underlies menopause problems and degenerative changes is without scientific validity, evidence or clinical back up.

The British Menopause Society's general warnings were soon followed by more specific ones from medical advisers to the National Osteoporosis Society. They insisted they could not recommend the use of 'natural progesterone' in any form either to prevent osteoporosis or to protect the womb if used instead of a regular progestogen in HRT. I would also emphasize that neither progesterone nor progestogen can offer protection against cardio-vascular disease as oestrogen can.

Progestogen, which is the synthetic form of progesterone, was developed because natural progesterone is too quickly 'used up' in the body and, in a dose sufficient to protect the womb lining, tends to make women very sleepy. Although progesterone *gel* has not undergone controlled trials (and British gynaecologists have been informed that none are planned) trials are being carried out with natural progesterone as nasal sprays or vaginal pessaries. These may occasionally be prescribed at the discretion of individual doctors, as part of HRT used instead of a progestogen, but only in a controlled setting and usually as part of a trial.

Perhaps the most exciting finding in recent years regarding HRT has been that it also protects against strokes and heart attacks, as well as protecting bone.

It had been suspected for a long time that oestrogen was beneficial to the cardio-vascular system, but in the last few years several authoritative American studies have confirmed that HRT given after the menopause positively protects the heart and arteries.[7]

The circumstantial evidence for oestrogen being involved in heart protection has always been pretty convincing. There was the fact that during our fertile years, when oestrogen levels are high, women rarely have heart attacks. In contrast, of course, the records show young men under forty being at least twenty times more prone to this problem than women of comparable age.[8]

Then, after the menopause, when oestrogen production drops, women rapidly lose their built-in advantage. In the forty- to forty-nine-year age group, the male to female heart attack ratio drops from twenty to one to only three to one; and in the fifty- to fifty-nine-year age group it goes down to two to one, where it eventually levels out.

It was also clearly significant that quite young women who had their ovaries removed and inevitably became oestrogen deficient, developed higher blood-cholesterol levels than controls of comparable age, *and* developed four times the risk of heart disease. This ruled out age itself as a major factor in the disease.[9]

Cholesterol, as everyone knows, is the blood fat most closely associated with a predisposition to heart attacks, and clinical studies have found that high cholesterol levels in men, especially in the younger age groups, appear to be related to the development of coronary artery disease.

Doctors have believed for a long time that lack of oestrogen after the ovaries fail, or are removed, could be responsible, at least in part, for increased levels of cholesterol and increased incidence of cardio-vascular disease. If that were the case, it would be logical that replacing oestrogen should bring cholesterol levels down. This is precisely what was found when checks were done on women using HRT.[10]

However, the influence of oestrogen turned out to be even more beneficial than just reducing *overall* cholesterol. In recent years, *two* types of cholesterol have been found to be at work. One called low density lipoprotein (LDL) is the real 'baddy' acting to *deposit* fat in the arteries. The other high density lipoprotein (HDL), is the 'goody' helping to scour fat deposits out. Oestrogen has been found not only to *reduce* the harmful LDL, but to *increase* levels of beneficial HDL.

This helps to explain the extraordinary protection which the American work found that HRT exerted on heart and arteries, *reducing cardio-vasular disease by 50 per cent.*[11]

Now, however, because most of these studies were based on use of oestrogen alone, it has become vital for further research to be done to ensure the progestogen content of *combined* HRT (used routinely today for women with a womb to protect) does not undermine the protective effect of oestrogen on the heart.

So efforts are currently concentrated on identifying the type of progestogen that will cause the least disturbance to the beneficial HDL/LDL ratio induced by oestrogen, but at the same time continue to give full protection to the womb lining. Sorting this out and developing new progestogens to even better fulfil these requirements has become a priority. The discovery that HRT can reduce to such a degree mortality rates from heart attacks and strokes has given it new importance and status. Today, with this tremendous reinforcement of the advantages of this treatment over any risks, even the most anti-HRT doctors have been forced to re-think.

Other forms of long-term protection continue to emerge from ongoing trials. Preventing bone loss has also been found to prevent loosening of teeth and to help maintain healthy gums. It is also increasingly recognized that HRT preserves muscle tone and helps prevent incontinence, that most dreaded symptom of old age.[12]

Among elderly ladies, on both sides of the Atlantic, HRT has also been found to have a beneficial effect on uterine prolapse. In some cases, it restores tone so well to pelvic supporting structures that the need for surgery is obviated.

Where controlled trials have been carried out, it has also been found that elderly patients receiving oestrogen tend to become less apathetic and more interested in life than untreated patients.[13]

Similar results were reported by a pioneering British doctor, John Maddison, as long ago as the 1960s. He had become convinced of the value of HRT when running a geriatric centre at Teddington, and carried out trials over a fifteen-year period. Dr Maddison told me,

We observed the clinical state of some 2000 old people,

taking regular checks for height, strength of hand-grip, mental ability and so on. Among the women, half were given oestrogen and half were not. Those on oestrogen replacement showed no loss of height, while among the others there was up to two inches in loss over the same period, due to osteoporosis. The ones on oestrogen also kept happier and more alert.

The tonic effect of oestrogen on mental as well as physical symptoms has been reaffirmed since by numerous studies, but one new American trial reported when I was visiting the States in 1993, went further. It indicated that replacing oestrogen might delay onset of Alzheimer's and the severe memory loss this inflicts.

That original study was carried out in a retirement complex in California and involved 8879 elderly women. Doctors found that those receiving oestrogen proved 40 per cent less likely to develop Alzheimer's than those *not* receiving it, with higher doses of oestrogen appearing to offer greater protection.[13]

The existence of oestrogen-binding sites in the brain has been known for some time, but the actual mechanism by which oestrogen protects against loss of the brain cells involved in Alzheimer's is not fully understood. Doctors believe the answer lies, at least in part, with oestrogen increasing the blood supply to the brain.

The American results have sparked tremendous further studies worldwide, including some very interesting work under way at King's College Hospital, London. Dr Malcolm Whitehead, the consultant gynaecologist who heads the Menopause Clinic there, told me that they are comparing brain scans of women over the age of sixty to check for differences between those on HRT and those who are not.

'The evidence that HRT may help to protect against Alzheimer's is so important that it must be investigated to the full,' he told me. 'If the American study is backed by others, then we are facing an important medical breakthrough offering real hope that HRT may provide some defence against a cruelly disabling condition, which takes as a heavy toll on sufferers, their carers and the NHS.'

So yet another form of long-term oestrogen protection may be in view. All of them have their special importance. Heart disease can kill, osteoporosis can cripple *and* kill, and even the common and undignified incontinence can make life a misery both for the elderly victim, who is often depressed and ashamed, and for the relatives or nurses who have to cope with it.

But there is one form of possible long-term protection not yet mentioned. Although osteoporosis kills more women than ovarian cancer and cervical cancer put together, and heart disease remains the biggest killer of all, it is cancer that women fear most. And so in the next chapter we shall be looking at evidence for the view taken by a consensus of leading doctors. On balance, modern HRT is actually *protective* against cancer.

Chapter 5

Protection against cancer?

In science and in medicine one finding leads to another, one set of observations suggests a further line or enquiry. It was in this way that Dr Gordan in San Francisco made the startling discovery that oestrogen appeared to have some protective role against cancer. In the follow-up of women on long-term cyclic oestrogen treatment for osteoporosis, he found there was an unexpected and significant reduction in the incidence of all forms of cancer.[1]

Similar reports began to come from other independent studies, and as long ago as January 1971, that august and cautious medical paper, *The Lancet*, drew attention to these findings, quoting four studies involving 1130 female patients, all treated with cyclic oestrogen for between five and seventeen years. The normal expected number of cancers should have been seventy-six. There were two.

In another study of 1422 women, made by Professor John Bakke, some ninety-six cases of cancer would have been expected to show up, and only five did. In a further study, 292 patients, also on long-term oestrogen, revealed *no* cases of breast cancer at all, when statistically there should have been sixteen.[2]

One of the most intriguing retrospective studies was completed just before I went over to America to research for the first edition of this book, and I went to see the authors, Drs John Burch and Benjam Byrd, who were working at Vanderbilt University School of Medicine in Nashville, Tennessee. The two men had carried out a 100 per cent follow-up of 713 patients, ranging in age from twenty-seven to eighty-five. All these women had undergone a hysterectomy at some time between 1948 and 1967, and all had received continuous oestrogen therapy from shortly after surgery onwards.

The study set out to look at three things in particular: the incidence of breast cancer; the incidence of all forms of cancer; and the general mortality rate.

The results of the study were so startling that they were subjected to the most careful scrutiny available, both medically and statistically. No criticism could be found, and in all cases figures had been corrected to allow for the hysterectomies having eliminated the risk of uterine cancer.

Briefly, the survey showed that although the number of breast cancer cases in the group was comparable to that anticipated in any group of women of the same ages, in the oestrogen-treated women, these cases came ten years later.[3]

The real surprise, however, was the finding that the incidence of *all* cancers showed a steady decline, with only *one-third* of the anticipated incidence in *oestrogen-treated* women aged forty and over. Most dramatic of all, *after* the age of forty-five, the mortality rate in treated women dropped to *half* that expected in women of comparable ages. Studies that have taken place since have failed to find the same 'delay effect' of oestrogen treatment on breast cancer development, but they *have* confirmed the 50 per cent reduction in overall mortality rates in women on HRT. Also figures from on-going epidemiological studies being carried out in Oxford[4] confirm mortality rates for breast cancer are significantly *reduced* in women on HRT.

Despite this, the breast cancer position remains confused. Although the Oxford research indicates mortality rate down, the actual incidence of breast cancer appears to be slightly higher in women after ten years on HRT, rising from the normal one in fifteen women to one in twelve. Some other studies show a similar small, but significant increase and yet these are completely contradicted by several far larger studies that have found *less* breast cancer in women on HRT.

One example was quoted at the International Menopause Symposium in Rome, in 1979. There, Dr Kirby Bland presented the findings of the Louisville Breast Cancer Detection Demonstration Project. That long title covers an equally long survey, involving data on 14,023 patients. From these, over 400 patients were selected for whom there were *complete* hormonal and mammographical histories. All were post-menopausal (natural or surgical), and all were between the ages of thirty-seven and eighty-four, with a mean age of 59.7. These were group-matched precisely by age, number of children and presence or absence of breast symptoms, together with use or non-use of oestrogen. The results showed a 'negative' association – that is, the number of patients with cancer among *non-users* of HRT was higher than among actual users – 9.0 per cent against 3.4 per cent.[5]

Very similar results, showing breast cancer again reduced by one-third in women on HRT, were reported by Dr Gambrell in his full-scale studies carried out in Texas.[6] One of the most reassuring studies, reported in the *American Journal of Epidemiology*, came late in 1995. This compared 3130 post-menopausal women with diagnosed breast cancer with 3698 healthy women, finding *no* evidence of HRT influencing risk. No increased incidence of the disease was found in women who had ever used the treatment, and no significant increase showed up even among the small number of patients on HRT for more than fifteen years.[7]

Despite these latest findings, at the moment it is not possible to draw any firm conclusions. Apart from contradictory results, there are a lot of complicating factors that have to be taken into account. For instance, many women included in published studies did not start out on the *combined* HRT, which is routinely prescribed today when a woman has a womb to protect. So this raises the question of whether the inclusion of ten to twelve days' progestogen alongside oestrogen in each cycle may have a protective effect on the breast, similar to the one it has on the womb lining?

Again, does the fact that women on HRT often get better medical supervision account for more breast cancers being diagnosed in this group in some studies? And, if so, are they also detected earlier? And does this help explain the lower mortality rate?

Unfortunately, because cancer of the breast has a long latent period, it may be many years before results start feeding through from enough women, whose entire HRT experience has been on the combined therapy, to allow these questions to be fully answered.

Although consensus medical opinion today advises that for maximum insurance against any possible increased breast cancer risk, HRT should be limited to eight or ten years, the overall balance of risk and benefit still comes down heavily in favour of long-term treatment.

At a medical meeting, where I was speaking, Dr Klim McPherson of the Epidemiological Unit in Oxford summed up the present position well, when he gave the following advice to over 400 GPs present – a turn-out which reflected the massive current interest in this whole subject. He told them, 'The advantages of HRT are so powerful and enormous that although one should not ignore any disadvantages, one should get them into balance and let women decide for themselves.'

This book is designed to help you do that, providing you with all the current information. And this needs to cover the position with regard to uterine cancer.

Experts on both sides of the Atlantic always warned that there might be some increased risk of this disease if oestrogen was used, on its own, over prolonged periods for women who still had a womb. This was because although oestrogen does not make a woman fertile again after the menopause, it does do its old job of building up the lining of the womb as if there really could be a fertilized egg to implant.

If this build-up of lining is not regularly shed – as pioneers of HRT like Dr Robert Wilson in America and Sir John Peel, in Britain all recognized – there could be at least a hypothetical risk of unhealthy thickening taking place. This condition, called hyperplasia, was known to exist with or precede uterine cancer, and there were fears that in a few cancer-prone women it might offer a pathway to uterine cancer.

The obvious way to guard against this is to give HRT in a form that simulates the natural protective hormone pattern. This would then guarantee the womb lining is regularly and completely shed just as it is each month during our fertile life.

For this to happen, the ovaries must first produce oestrogen and then, in the second half of each cycle, the other female sex hormone, progesterone. Progesterone further modifies the womb lining, ready for any egg to implant, but if no conception takes place, levels of both hormones drop. It is the fall in progesterone, however, that provides the really powerful trigger that induces the womb lining to shed, taking with it the unfertilized egg in the monthly flow that we call menstruation.

To achieve the same safe and protective shedding on HRT, experts insisted a progestrogen (the oral form of progesterone) should be given alongside oestrogen for the last part of each cycle.

It was the obvious and safe answer but, unfortunately, was not always used in America. Women in America can dictate the treatment they want to their doctors in a way that we cannot here, and feeling so well on oestrogen many saw the addition of progestogen as a complication, especially since it involved an obligatory bleed.

Under threat of cheque books being taken elsewhere, and no doubt because at the time it *was* only a vague hypothetical risk, many American physicians fell back on what they believed to be a safe compromise. They prescribed oestrogen alone, but on a cyclical basis, three weeks on and one week off. In the week off treatment, it was *assumed* that the fall in oestrogen would be sufficient in itself to trigger shedding of any womb lining that might have built up. If no bleed occurred, it was again *assumed* there was no build-up.

This proved over-optimistic, and wrong on all counts. In 1975, the alarm bells rang across America, as simultaneous retrospective studies were published showing the hypothetical risk was all too real. Small but significant increases in uterine cancer had been found in women on oestrogen therapy.

Fortunately, the same thing did not happen in this country. It is to the credit of British medicine that it was not content to deal in hypothetical risks or theoretical protection. Well before the American scare, three of our leading menopause clinics had already started sampling the womb lining of every patient coming for treatment, both before and after different regiments of HRT. This work confirmed that on oestrogen alone, even given on a cyclical basis, a few women did develop hyperplasia. In every case, the condition regressed completely on treatment with progestogen. More to the point, the British work also established that progestogen used alongside oestrogen for ten to twelve consecutive days each month gave maximum protection – no hyperplasia occurred, and there was no increased risk of uterine cancer.[8]

This British research set firm guidelines for safe administration of HRT, which have since been accepted worldwide. For any woman who has a womb to protect, use of the combined therapy is now considered mandatory, and this system had proved to add to the cancer protection that HRT gives. Results feeding through from monitoring thousands of women on this treatment show that combined HRT does not just eliminate the increased risk of uterine cancer that can occur on oestrogen alone, it actually *reduces* the normal risk, with the incidence of this disease *cut by half in women on treatment*.

Many doctors also believe that HRT protects against cancer of the ovaries. This is because every case-controlled study of the oral contraceptive has found the Pill to protect against ovarian cancer, with the incidence again reduced by half. Logically, therefore, HRT should exert the same protective influence, and studies are being done to test this.

Where cervical cancer is concerned, repeated studies have failed to find any increase in this disease on HRT. A history of successfully treated cervical cancer is *not* considered a contra-indication for HRT.

The fact that a history of other forms of cancer usually precludes a woman being put on HRT has sometimes been mistakenly interpreted as suggesting that HRT is actually implicated in inducing cancer. The position in reality is that excluding women who have had cancer is just a precaution against the existence of secondary tumours, a possibility that must be reckoned with in such cases. Because oestrogen stimulates the growth of certain types of cells, including malignant ones of the same sort (if they *should* be present), it is thought safer to avoid any chance of this happening. This rule is being increasingly relaxed where menopause problems are acute, where heart disease or osteoporosis already exist, or where there is a high risk of either.

Despite the fact that HRT has been shown to be protective in certain types of cancer, a great deal more work needs to be done before claims that it gives *general* cancer protection can be justified. As most people today realize, cancer is a condition of undisciplined cell division rather than a single disease, and it almost certainly has many different causes.

However, the indications for oestrogen's general ability to exert a beneficial influence are strong. In fact, there is growing clinical and statistical evidence of the protective role of oestrogen in regard to many forms of disease, and more and more research is being directed towards finding the mechanism at work.

One man, whose life-time study of the body's defence system throws some possible light on this, is Thomas Nicol, Professor of Anatomy at King's College, London, for thirty-one years. He told me:

More than thirty years of research and thousands of experiments have provided convincing proof that oestrogen is a natural stimulant of the body's defences against infection, premature ageing and certain forms of cancer. It is the petrol that fuels the whole defence system.

Our experiments have shown that oestrogen stimulates the white cells of the blood and increases their power to mop up invading organisms. This ability of oestrogen to activate the defence mechanism explains why men do not generally live as long as women, whose bodies consistently produce more oestrogen. It also explains why pregnant women, who have high oestrogen levels, are usually healthier and less liable to infection. Further, it explains the fact that depression, fear and worry are able to lower resistance, and damage the body's defences, almost certainly through a feed-back mechanism affecting hormone balance.[9]

Fortunately the technique of radioimmunoassay, which now enables us to measure hormone levels in the blood accurately, makes it possible to rectify the hormone imbalances which come with ageing. The essential problem now is to establish healthy norms, the baseline from which to work.

This is very much the way in which HRT should ideally be used, with the individual normal hormone levels for each woman established *before* the onset of the menopause causes them to drop. With limited resources, this is not practical at the moment, but tailoring the *type* of HRT and *dosage* to individual need is very much the state of the art in good prescription practice today.

Meanwhile, with the short-term advantages so clearly

obvious, and the long-term protective role against osteoporosis and cardio-vascular disease so well proven, women are entitled to ask *why* British medicine has taken so long to officially endorse HRT. Even more perplexing is why it was ever considered so controversial. Even back in the 1970s when I first started campaigning, Hormone Replacement was already the indicated and widely used treatment for all other hormone deficiency states – thyroid, adrenal, diabetes, etc. Yet there was massive resistance to the logical extension of this concept to counter the oestrogen deficiency that follows the menopause.

So why was the menopause felt to be different? And what were the objections that doctors raised in the past and to which a few of them still obstinately cling? The next chapter provides some of the answers.

Chapter 6

The medical controversy

It was when my research took me round British medical schools that I began to understand the basis for the resistance that doctors showed in this country to the concept of HRT. Not only in the 1970s was this treatment entirely absent from the syllabus, but medical students were still being firmly taught that because sooner or later ovarian failure occurs in *all* women, it must be considered natural and therefore requiring no treatment.

Universality seemed to me a poor reason for non-treatment, and one certainly not applied to the other degenerative changes that come with age – failing sight, declining hearing or decaying teeth! These aspects of ageing, of course, are common to both sexes, while the menopause is a purely female matter and, as such, could presumably be written off as just another unfortunate little quirk of nature that women had 'to put up with'. After all, their mothers had sweated their way through it – and their grandmothers too – so what was all the fuss about now?

That seemed to be the attitude of most doctors I talked to in the early days and, no doubt, within the then largely male-dominated medical profession of those days, it was considered a perfectly reasonable stance. It was certainly a convenient one, perhaps even justifiable when no really effective treatment existed. But in 1973 it *did* exist. HRT had by then been used successfully elsewhere in the world to correct oestrogen deficiency problems for over a decade.

The prevailing attitude was described to me by one doctor as 'benign neglect'. 'That means if we are doing no good,' he explained, 'at least we are doing no harm'. He was utterly wrong. That 'benign neglect' was dooming thousands of women unnecessarily not merely to temporary menopause miseries but, in many cases, also to the permanent, grim legacy left by failing ovaries. While the effectiveness of HRT in protecting against heart disease and strokes had not then been proven, there was already solid evidence showing that it prevented accelerated bone loss at the menopause and prevented osteoporosis.

So while doctors might argue that flushes were natural, and never killed anyone, they could hardly argue the same for osteoporotic fractures. Of course, the full extent of that problem was not fully recognized back in the 1970s, and certainly the vast majority of women remained completely unaware of any connection between loss of oestrogen and the bent backs, pain and fractures they might experience later in life.

They *were* aware, however, of the more obvious and immediate problems the menopause could bring, and some women proved desperate enough to consult their doctors despite general medical apathy on the subject. To be fair, where this happened, a few of the more compassionate GPs did try to help with symptomatic treatment. They would prescribe Valium or Librium for depression, which only served to make it rather worse, and pain killers for backache and headache which only brought temporary relief. But the majority of women who dared to complain were simply dismissed with a pat on the shoulder and the dreaded words: 'It's just your age. You must put up with it'.

The one place where I discovered women did *not* have to 'put up with it' was in the private sector. For any woman who could afford to knock on the doors of Harley Street, it seemed the menopause was not so natural after all. I found the top specialists already knew a great deal about HRT, and used it widely for their patients, not just for several months but for several years, clearly recognizing the protection it afforded against brittle bones in the longer term.

It was there that I met Sir John Peel, then the Queen's own gynaecologist. Luckily for all of us, he believed, as I did, that HRT should not just remain privileged medicine, but be available for any woman who needed and wanted it. It was the public support Sir John gave me, in allowing me to quote him in articles and programmes, and eventually in writing the Foreword for this book, that helped to give HRT the respectability it so badly needed at that time.

But even with his help, and the pioneering efforts of a few early enthusiasts among British gynaecologists, it was still a long time before British medicine began to accept that HRT was not just some new-fangled import from America, (designed to make money), but a treatment that could be usefully employed under the NHS, and within general practice.

The younger doctors, as might be expected, were the most open-minded and ready to at least try out replacement therapy. Where they did not already know much about it, some, like my own GP, took the trouble to read up on it. Once this was done, they usually began to prescribe, only cautiously at first, for severe menopause problems, but later, gaining confidence with each success, they became converted to wider usage.

The GPs' attitudes in any one area tended to stem from the top, with the leading gynaecologists' known views exerting considerable influence. In one big city, where at the time HRT was particularly hard to get, the Professor of Obstetrics and Gynaecology told me flatly, 'I am horrified at the idea of looking at the menopause as a disease. This kind of thinking is for the birds, and for those in private practice who have time on their hands, where, no doubt it will prove a gold mine.'

Having gone on to condemn HRT as unnecessary in anything but very small doses, to relieve very acute symptoms, he made one final somewhat surprising concession. He added, 'I would say if a menopausal woman marries again, she *should* have oestrogen replacement as it keeps the vagina young.' Presumably, women still on Mark 1 husbands and marriages can just struggle on with old vaginas!

In fairness, I must add that this particular consultant, despite personal lack of enthusiasm for replacement therapy, still allowed John Studd, then a young registrar on his professiorial unit, to set up one of the first NHS menopause clinics in this country.

These special clinics began to proliferate in the mid-1970s, in direct response to the increasing pressure from women for menopause treatment. As they learned through the press and media that HRT existed, understood its logic and saw its benefits, women were no longer prepared to 'put up with it', and doctors' surgeries were besieged.

Not surprisingly, a lot of GPs felt unable to prescribe something they knew almost nothing about. So, to help meet the demand for HRT, a chain of NHS menopause clinics was set up. These served a double purpose, acting as referral centres to which doctors could send menopausal patients, and also serving as research centres where much-needed studies could be carried out with a ready supply of ladies happy to take part in monitoring programmes.

As Sir John Peel points out in his Foreword to this book, there were many controversial aspects of HRT which badly needed sorting out at that time. Some offered more valid cause for concern than others, but reassurance was sought on all of them before doctors were prepared to accept that HRT was safe.

There was never any question about the treatment being effective. At the twentieth British Congress of Obstetrics and Gynaecology in 1974, the Birmingham menopause clinic reported HRT giving 100 per cent control of hot flushes in their special trials, and they also confirmed its protective role over the skeletal system.[1]

The rapid elimination of flushes, sweats and vaginal atrophy, of course, was something that GPs could readily confirm for themselves. Long-term safety was a different matter.

The first fear they expressed about this was in connection with increased thrombosis risk. Studies had only recently shown this to be associated with use of the contraceptive Pill, and in Britain doctors were quick to wrongly extrapolate a similar risk to HRT on the basis that both involved use of oestrogen and progestogen.

Through the medical press and menopause symposia designed to update doctors on menopause management, the differences between HRT and the Pill were made clear. Firstly, the Pill *adds* to existing hormone levels, while HRT, as the name implies, merely *replaces* missing hormones.

But the main difference, perhaps needing even more emphasis since the 1996 report showing some increased thrombosis risk on certain low-dose Pills, is that HRT only requires such a small amount of oestrogen (one-eighth of that contained in even the lowest-dose birth-control Pill) that an entirely different type of oestrogen can be used. Unlike the Pill, HRT can be based on very small doses of *natural* oestrogen – that is oestrogen of the same type that the ovaries themselves produce.

In contrast, the Pill must employ very much higher doses to actually inhibit ovulation, and this means using powerful *synthetic* oestrogens. It is these which have been associated with increased incidence of thrombosis. Repeated studies have failed to find any evidence of *natural* oestrogen ever causing this problem.

Thrombosis risk is closely linked to blood-clot potential, and as long ago as 1968, *The Lancet* published work showing that while synthetic oestrogen *did* adversely affect the behaviour of blood constituents called 'platelets', increasing their stickiness and clotting potential, natural oestrogen did not have the same effect and nor did progestogens when tested.[2] Since then many other studies have confirmed this.[3]

More understandable than any worries over thrombosis, were the fears many doctors harboured of some link between oestrogens and cancer. They muttered darkly about that 'stilbestrol business', and certainly it was that particular tragedy, surfacing as it did so inopportunely in 1971, that helped create a distinctly anti-oestrogen climate.

Stilbestrol had been officially classed as a 'synthetic' oestrogen, but the distinction between synthetic and natural oestrogens was not well understood in those days. In actual fact, stilbestrol is a coal-tar derivative, and cannot properly be described as an oestrogen at all, although it possesses oestrogenic properties – that is, it performs some of the functions of an oestrogen. In particular, it helps to prevent miscarriages and to rid the body of milk after pregnancy. It is also both effective and cheap, with the result that it was widely used for both those purposes and sometimes even to treat acute menopausal problems.

Back in the 1930s, in the early days of cancer and hormone research, which developed together, many substances had been tried out for cancer-producing properties, and one of them was stilbestrol. Massive amounts were given to laboratory-bred mice and tumours developed. As coal-tar derivatives are now known carcinogens, this was not really surprising, especially as the mice were a special cancer-prone strain, and were fed half their own body-weight of stilbestrol over a six-month period, which represents about one quarter of their normal life span.

It has been estimated that a woman would have to swallow about 150 pounds of stilbestrol over half her lifetime to receive a comparable dose.[4] Experiments done at the same time to produce similar tumours, by feeding stilbestrol to mice belonging to a strain in which spontaneous breast cancer in females seldom occurred, entirely failed. In fact, all further experiments since then, feeding oestrogens to mice, rats and, even more relevantly, to monkeys over a ten-year period, had failed to reproduce any forms of cancer.[5]

But fears regarding stilbestrol were freshly aroused in 1971, when reports began to come in from the New England area in America, that a proportion of female offspring of women treated with stilbestrol some twenty years earlier to prevent miscarriage, had developed vaginal cancers after puberty. By 1974, an appalling total of 170 young girls had been found to be affected, and this was reported in the *American Journal of Obstetrics and Gynaecology.*[6]

It added up to a terrible tragedy but, significantly, there was no case in which the mother herself developed any form of cancer. It was a clear example, and a terrible one, of the extreme vulnerability of the foetus to hormone influence, with puberty probably supplying a second hormone trigger.

A top American gynaecologist and endocrinologist, Professor Robert Greenblatt, with whom I discussed this, explained: 'Stilbestrol clearly crossed the placental barrier and the foetal liver could not metabolize it. It serves to point its clear difference to natural oestrogen, because mothers have colossal amounts of that in their bodies during pregnancy and the foetus is unharmed.'

The full lesson to be learned, of course, is that stilbestrol should never be used to treat a pregnant woman, and certainly not for HRT. In fact, with such a wide choice of natural oestrogens now available, there is no need for synthetic oestrogens to be used at all for menopause management. Details of HRT products containing natural oestrogen are included in Chapter 10.

In the minds of some doctors, fear of a link between hormones and cancer also arose from the fact that some forms of breast cancer can be what is termed 'hormone dependent'; that is, their cell growth is stimulated by oestrogen. At one time, it was not unusual for the ovaries in such cases to be removed in an attempt to slow down progress of the disease. Today, a drug called tamoxifen makes this unnecessary.

As explained earlier, there is all the difference between stimulating the growth of existing cancer cells, and *causing* them in the first place, but this is not always sufficiently emphasized.

The one good reason for British doctors maintaining a cautious approach to HRT back in the 1970s was fear that prolonged use of oestrogen might result in increased risk of uterine cancer. As we have seen, there were at least some grounds for this both in theory and, after the publication of the American findings published in 1975, also in practice.

Appendix 3 gives fuller details of these American studies, and of the result of conversations I had with Dr Smith, the author of the biggest of them, regarding the actual cancer classifications. When he revealed these it certainly seemed to our experts here that a great deal of the so-called cancer was in fact only reversible hyperplasia, and that possibly, fear of litigation and a degree of hype in the press had exaggerated the scare.

Fortunately, the British work, proving the protective nature of combined HRT, came at exactly the right time to short-circuit another repetition of the problem here. Today, no doctor who keeps up with the literature can any longer raise the spectre of uterine cancer as an objection to HRT. On the contrary, we know that the therapy reduces its incidence by half.[7]

Another fear expressed by some doctors, that the combined system of HRT helped to overcome, was that breakthrough bleeding could mask post-menopausal bleeding from a more sinister cause. They had a valid point, but fortunately, using the combined therapy, the monthly withdrawal bleed always comes at the planned and scheduled time, usually within forty-eight hours of the progestogen course being completed. This means that unexpected and suspect bleeding can be identified and investigated.

While this system of regular withdrawal bleeds, as we saw in America, is not always popular with patients, studies in our NHS menopause clinics have shown that if the vital protective purposes are explained, 90 per cent of women will accept it.

Within any structure of socialized, free or insured medicine, economic arguments and comparisons of priority needs are bound to be heard. There were dire prophecies in the early days about the extra time and expense that would be involved if mass demand for HRT was encouraged.

In practice, doctors prescribing HRT have found that it actually costs far less than the Librium and Valium once dished out so uselessly to menopausal women, and they also discovered that in the end it saved on doctor hours by eliminating consultations in the short term, for common menopause conditions such as flushes and depression, and in the long term, for more serious problems against which HRT protects.

The latest – excellent – trend is for GPs to offer menopause treatment as part of the services within a weekly Well Woman clinic. In Japan, industry set an interesting example in economics, with one large firm coming down in favour of HRT, and providing it free at their own medical centre, as a means of cutting down on absenteeism among menopausal women employees.

With medical fears overcome and initial much-toted economic objections hardly sustainable in view of HRT's proven ability to reduce costs incurred in treatment of heart disease, strokes and osteoporosis, it is amazing that any doctor can still refuse treatment or parrot old outdated objections. Yet organizations like Women's Health Concern, a charity that for nearly a quarter of a century has promoted menopause education and treatment, confirms that this does happen. Joan Jenkins who founded and runs WHC told me, 'Although things have improved, we still get letters from some women whose doctors refuse them HRT and will only give them tranquillizers. Despite all we now know, there are even a few doctors who still insist the menopause is natural and women must sweat it out. In our experience HRT provision is patchy, and even today some women may need to stand up for their right to receive the correct and appropriate replacement therapy. One of our jobs is to educate and inform women so that they have the confidence to do this.'

Joan feels, as I do, that if men suffered an abrupt physical menopause in mid-life, with atrophy of sex organs, falling hormone levels, and failing libido, we should have heard very little about it all being natural. HRT would have been instituted a long time ago.

So just how natural is the female menopause? What purpose does it serve? And why is the human female the only one in all of nature to go through the 'change of life'.

Chapter 7

The menopause and evolution

In the whole of nature, only the human female suffers a physical menopause. While other animals remain potentially fertile until death, a woman is deliberately programmed for her ovaries to shut down in mid-life. When the number of eggs stored in the ovaries has declined to a certain level, new orders are triggered for the ovaries to cease to produce oestrogen. Finally they atrophy and shrivel, bringing an end to her fertile life.

The age at which this usually happens has always been between forty-five and fifty. Aristotle, who lived over three hundred years before Christ, wrote, '... for the most part fifty marks the limit of women's reproductive capacity'. Avicenna, a famous Arab physician of the eleventh century, pointed out: 'There are women whose menopause lapses quickly to end in their thirty-fifth or fortieth year, but there are others in whom it lasts until they reach fifty'.

There are many fantastic claims of late fertility, including the biblical story of Sarah bearing a child when over ninety. However, such reports from ancient times and civilizations where births and deaths were not officially registered as they are today are notoriously unreliable. If we exclude results of modern fertility treatment, the oldest, fully documented birth was to Mrs Ruth Alice Kistler of America, who is reported in the *Guinness Book of Records* as giving birth to a daughter in 1956, at the age of fifty-seven years, 129 days.

At the other end of the scale, some women do suffer

a very early menopause in the thirties, and occasionally ovarian failure may occur even before that.

Extensive records show that the age at which these fresh instructions begin to operate, and the date of final menstruation, are closely linked in mothers and daughters, a fact which tends to confirm the genetic nature of the control of the underlying process. Instances of premature menopause in the same family provide the most striking evidence of this. In one family three sisters are recorded ceasing menstruation at thirty-three, thirty-eight and thirty-three respectively, and their mother at forty-two.

It is interesting that modern records are now showing the average age for the menopause extended to over fifty-one, and with puberty also coming earlier, it would appear to indicate adaptation to the longer life-span by an extension also of female fertile life.

But why is the female blueprint designed in this particular way to set a limit of fertility? Why did evolution favour the female menopause in the human race? And why are women unique in this respect?

The reasons seem clear, if somewhat negative. The most important advantage was ensuring that ova which had been stored too long had no chance to be fertilized. There is a tendency for ova to deteriorate over the years and an example of this is the higher incidence of mongolism in babies born to older mothers, due to defective chromosomes in the female egg.

In contrast male sperm is not stored and is not, therefore, subject to the same risk of deterioration. It is freshly manufactured throughout life.

Another reason for limiting the period of fertility in women was to ensure that children should not be born in mothers unlikely to live long enough to rear them. The human child is dependent on its mother for many years, and in the past repeated and dangerous childbearing, lack of hygiene, poor nutrition and little medical knowledge meant that women died young. It seems incredible today to realize that at the time of the

Roman Empire the average life expectancy for a woman was only twenty-five. By the time of the discovery of America it had increased to about thirty years, and even by the Victorian era it had only risen to forty-five.

Another and more subtle reason for the menopause, put forward by one anthropologist, was the need to ensure some older women surviving to pass on acquired female wisdom and skills. By eliminating the special hazards of late childbirth, there was an improved chance of a few old wise women living on to the benefit of both tribe and race. In such primitive times the only means of passing on knowledge was by example, demonstration or word of mouth. The 'elders' of a tribe had a special status and special services to render.

So in evolutionary terms it can be seen that the menopause had an important part to play. But it was important to the individual woman too. It brought the only relief then known from the tyranny of constant pregnancies. Some wit once declared that the safest form of contraception has always been the word 'No' spoken firmly, but in rougher and ruder times, when women were merely possessions and wealth was counted in the number of sons, refusal had little effect on men who did not need to bother about the finer points of courtship or consent.

So, in the past, those women living beyond the menopause must have been mainly conscious of relief that the annual ordeal of childbirth appeared to be over.

The train of events that followed, the adverse effects on energy, health and appearance, were simply accepted as an inevitable part of ageing. Nature clearly lost interest in the infertile woman and saw no purpose in keeping her desirable, so the lack of oestrogen not only ended reproduction, but ended the positive effects on skin, muscle and bone, allowing accelerated ageing to take place.

Alongside the compensation of being free of child-bearing, a woman who survived beyond mid-life had to accept that she was old and had ceased to be sexually interesting. The menopause marked the end of her life as a desirable woman, and, since she could no longer produce sons, it also reduced her value as a wife.

One can imagine clear elements of personal tragedy in this for women, but for men it did not matter much. A man might get through several wives in the course of his life-time. His virility continued; he could go on enjoying sexual adventures and fathering children right into old age. He did not even have to bother about retaining youthful good looks and figure. This was not demanded as part of male attraction, as it was (and still is) demanded as part of female attraction. So the extraordinary double standards of behaviour and appearance, which we have come to take for granted, can be seen to be rooted to quite a large extent in the phenomena of the menopause, and in the striking contrast it produces in the way men and women age.

But because the majority of women did not survive long beyond the menopause anyway, and because it involved little or no inconvenience to the male, who had the money and power to decide the direction of any research, the menopause attracted little or no attention socially or medically until quite recently.

It is extraordinary looking through the literature on the subject to discover how little was really understood about the menopause and associated female phenomena until this century.

Because the menopause was seen as a negative thing, basically as the absence of the monthly 'issue of blood', folklore about it is inextricably linked with the mythology of menstruation, though assuming the opposite interpretations. So, to understand attitudes to the menopause, it is necessary to understand attitudes to menstruation.

In the very beginning, because blood was associated in the primitive mind with wounds, injuries and death, menstruation was viewed with fear and superstition. It became the subject of strict taboos in every culture, and there is still an echo of this in our own rational age in the lingering use of the old euphemism, 'the curse'.

Pliny, who lived from AD 23 to 79, wrote many books, among them one called *Natural History*, which has been described as the first encyclopaedia. In it he points out that menstruating women had disastrous effects on quite ordinary things. They not only turned wine sour and seeds sterile, but caused grass and garden plants to wither and fruit to fall from any tree beneath which they sat.

In ancient times menstruating women were so much objects of dread that in many cultures there was a prohibition against any contact with them, and in some parts of the world they were even segregated into special huts, built at some distance from the villages.

They were obliged to call attention to their condition by smearing bright-coloured dyes on their faces or wearing masks, and even calling out, 'Unclean, unclean'. In Mosaic law a woman had to be put apart for seven days at the time of menstruation, and anyone or anything she touched became equally contaminated.

It is no surprise to find Christianity inheriting these old beliefs and forbidding women to enter sacred buildings while menstruating. But the superstition also extended into commerce, with menstruating women forbidden to work in sugar refineries in France, as they were thought to turn the sugar black. In Mexico the same ban applied to women working in the silver mines, as they caused the ore to disappear, while in Indo-China no woman was employed in the opium industry for fear that menstruation would turn the opium bitter.

To us now it seems just ancient rubbish but the idea persisted strongly for centuries, and as recently as 1878 a physician wrote to the *British Medical Journal*, reporting two instances where hams had been spoiled because a menstruating woman had cured them.

Until quite recently in some remote parts of England and Wales, it was still possible to find women being advised during menstruation not to touch red meat for fear it should 'go off', not to attempt to make bread because the dough would not rise, and never, never, for some inexplicable reason, to touch salt.

To the ancients the actual cause of menstruation was a complete mystery and it was blamed variously on gods, evil spirits, crocodiles, birds and the moon. The fact that it occurred at roughly four-week intervals strongly favoured the moon theory, and Aristotle asserted the moon was female because 'the menstrual flux and the waning of the moon both take place towards the end of the month, and after the wane and discharge both become whole again'.

The patent absurdity of a theory which would make all women menstruate at the same time seems to have worried very few people, and the superstition constantly reappeared. In 1704, no less a person than Richard Mead, physician to the English King, George II, wrote, 'In countries nearest the Equator where we have proved lunar action to be strongest, these monthly secretions are in much greater quantity than in those near the poles where the force is weakest'. Even more unbelievably, as recently as 1938, American medical students could still read in one of their most authoritative textbooks of obstetrics that 'over seventy-one per cent of women menstruate every twenty-eight days and the majority during the new moon'.

Although the moon was believed to have such influence in triggering the event, the purpose was widely believed to be a form of purging, by which women were relieved of impurities and excess blood. The belief that the flow contained poisonous material underlies more superstitions, and there is even, strangely, some modern support for this concept of a toxic substance, with women reporting that flowers fade, particularly if worn in a corsage, during the menstrual period. The theory put forward is that this toxic substance at such times also invades the perspiration.

Getting nearer the truth, but still vague and inaccurate, were the ideas of Hippocrates, the father of medicine, who at least groped towards the relationship between menstruation and reproduction with his theory that the menstrual flow was the nourishment which fed the child. Pliny went further, believing it was the actual substance from which the child was shaped and formed.

Whatever the view favoured, the opposite of menstruation, the cessation of the menstrual flow was still a bad thing. It meant that the woman was no longer getting rid of her 'evil humours' and the poisons were building up inside her, or it meant she no longer produced the substance of life. Either way she was diminished. She was no longer a real woman.

Margaret Mead, the famous American anthropologist, makes this point in her book, *Male and Female*. She found that both pre-pubertal girls and post-menopausal women in many societies were treated as men. Referring to the social role of women after the menopause, she writes,

Where reproductivity has been regarded as somewhat impure and ceremonially disqualifying – as in Bali – the post-menopausal woman and the virgin girl work together at ceremonies from which women of child-bearing age are debarred . . . Where modesty of speech and action is enjoined on women, such behaviour may no longer be asked from the older woman, who may use obscene language as freely as or more freely than any man.

This loss of femininity after the menopause and the change to neuter or masculine role is not only enshrined and emphasized by cultural attitudes and superstitions, but is something deeply felt by women, particularly the more uneducated and unsophisticated, whose role and status has been largely confined to the domestic and maternal. Such women vaguely envisage 'the change' as meaning real anatomical or structural changes taking place, and one seventy-year-old woman actually believed that women turned into men inside.

She insisted she had been aware of this process taking place and had felt it as a 'turning and tightening of the thigh muscles'.

In his excellent booklet *The Menopause – a neglected crisis*, Robert G. Richardson writes,

We must ask why an event of such significance to the individual woman passed almost without notice sociologically, anthropologically and medically. And the answer thrown back from the silent past is that the menopause was a negative event of no importance in the life of the community. So when a woman's usefulness was seen to be ended, she ceased to be a woman.

In the under-populated ancient world a woman's usefulness was measured by her fertility. In our modern crowded world the time is fast approaching when infertility in itself becomes a virtue. Certainly the fifty-plus woman today is no longer on the discard heap. Her wisdom, skill, experience and energy are badly needed and she becomes relatively 'young' in a population living to a new time-scale, which means that in Britain alone there are over nine million people aged over sixty-five.

Of course, with their conscious and reasoning minds women realize how much things have changed. They recognize their own value today to their families and to society. But beneath the surface old atavistic memories linger and lurk. And, amazing, as it may seem, some women today still give credence to dark notions that the menopause can cause them to lose their minds. They fear emotional and mental instability. Such a belief could be rooted in the very real evidence of depression and confusion which glandular imbalance can produce, but it almost certainly also stems from deeper hidden memories of a time when it was believed that the ageing female body could no longer expel the 'evil humours' in the cleansing monthly flux.

So science may banish superstition, modern medicine

eliminate the menopause, but old attitudes persist. Too many women still today feel diminished and threatened by the change of life. They fear not only mental and emotional instability, but actual sexual inadequacy, lack of response and loss of attraction.

It is fear of the castrating effect of the menopause plus the onset of emotional instability which, according to popular novels, drives previously respectable women to seek erotic adventures before the menopause robs them of all sexual satisfaction. In modern re-runs of this theme, it seems far more likely that today's authors would choose to invest such middle-aged female characters with the same sort of motivation that is ascribed to vulnerable middle-aged men: the need for reassurance that they are not yet over the hill and can still attract the opposite sex.

However, according to Dr Isobel Hutton, the middle-aged woman, hitherto of impeccable character, who goes off the rails, is not very true to life anyway. In her book, *The Hygiene of the Change in Women*, she writes,

Popular novels often give the impression that women are unduly amorous at this time and inclined to break loose from all decorum. We are familiar with the kind of literature in which women, at what is called 'the dangerous age', fall in love with young men and make themselves ridiculous with their overtures. These novels lead us to suppose that women are pursuing a last love affair before reaching the age which is supposed to be the end of their sex life.

In all the writer's experience, not a single case of this kind, directly attributable to the climacteric, has even been met with. An amorous, flighty woman will continue so throughout the 'change of life' and afterwards, but does not suddenly develop these characteristics between forty and fifty years of age.

If Isabel Hutton were writing today when toy-boys for the over-forties are much in fashion, she might be less sure of all this. But even if we accept that the onset of the menopause does not change a woman's basic moral values, it can certainly change her nature in other distinctly adverse ways. The letters I receive make it clear that many women at this time become irritable and difficult to live with. What is more, they are aware of this and worry about the effect on their family, but seem powerless to do anything about it. HRT helps by restoring hormonal balance, which in turn soothes the disturbed nervous system.

In his booklet on the menopause, Robert Richardson points out that not surprisingly, in view of their scientific interest during the nineteenth century, it was the French who incorporated these emotional aspects of the menopause into the literature of the period. He quotes from Octave Feuillet's comedy, *La Crise*, written in 1882. Julia, the heroine and a previously well-balanced personality, reflects:

What name can be given to this moral affliction, to this discontent with myself and with those about me that I have felt for some months. My husband, is doubtless, the best of men. But nothing that he says or does pleases me. His watch charms irritate me above all else. Yet these charms and I have lived together in peace for ten years. Then suddenly, one fine day, we hate each other. My husband has the insufferable habit of jingling them while he is talking – making an unbearable clinking. At the very instant that I write these lines he is in his room, winding his watch and making a noise with those charms.

Her husband, M. de Marsan, a magistrate, visits his doctor. He explains,

It is not a question of extravagant symptoms that would attract the attention of outsiders, but of shades, each day more marked, which do not escape an intimate like myself. For ten years I have said I possessed a treasure in my life. Then suddenly this sweet Julia takes on the air of a martyr – obedient, but irritated. This woman of the world, this refined woman now speaks a language full of sharp, bitter words, harsh and peevish maxims. I find in her conversation

– previously so mild – a banal melancholy, a sharp poetic flavour, with a socialist tendency which fills me with uneasiness . . . At the same time that the wife changed, the mother changed too. Her husband is now a tyrant, the children a heavy burden. She scarcely speaks to them. They are left to themselves. Here, then, doctor, is what happened to me. Here is the crown of thorns which Julia has put upon my innocent head, without the least provocation on my part. What is the explanation?

The doctor replies,

Perhaps I have it – your wife's age . . . It is a normal disease that may attack the best of women as they reach the threshold of maturity. Such is the attraction of the evil fruit which Eve held for the first time in her hands. Thus the most honoured woman may sense a desire not to be resigned to death without having tasted it.

Robert Richardson comments that thus, belatedly, both literature and medicine acknowledge that a woman's emotions are disturbed at the menopause and that, as Byron wrote in *Don Juan*, 'though her years were waning, her climacteric teased her like her teens'.

Chapter 8

The menopause and the modern family

The fact that both her family and society now accord the modern woman such an active and challenging role in middle age is far more a matter for congratulation than commiseration. To be thought young and to be encouraged to think of herself as young, is entirely on the credit side, but it does involve staying mentally and physically as fit as possible.

Some ten million post-menopausal women battling away in a world which makes little attempt to cushion them. Even if this were thought necessary, it would be difficult to achieve. The average family can neither afford nor obtain paid help, and the unpaid sort – once given by aunts, cousins and parents, usually just around the corner – has vanished along with the extended family. Our industrialized mobile society has brought not only dispersal of the family but the close-knit village community, once another source of support.

It has also brought a vast speeding up in communications, ideas and rates of change, so that the gap in thinking and attitudes between one generation and the next has widened to put the whole fabric of the family under stress. In the past, within the family and within society itself, roles and rules were sharply defined; parents were obeyed, elders respected and children protected. Each person knew his place, and few dared try to leave it or to question existing conditions and values. This whole safe, solid structure was firmly buttressed externally by the laws of church and state.

Today the middle-aged woman has no such certainties in her life and no simple rules either to live by herself, or to help her bring up her children. All authority is questioned and by the onset of menopause, she can find herself firmly stuck in a peculiar 'middle-aged sandwich', caught between worries over the adolescent children on one side, and problems starting to arise with her ageing parents on the other.

In addition to her complex role in the home, if she also does a full- or part-time job, she may well be facing extra problems at work as she reaches positions of greater responsibility.

In 1890, in America, only 6 per cent of married women worked. Today millions of women of forty-five or older, most of them married, are employed full-time, and some two-thirds of married women in all do paid or voluntary work.

The percentage of married women doing jobs in Great Britain is much the same, and so are their reasons for working. Apart from those who are officially registered as paid workers many more do small part-time jobs and voluntary welfare. Where once the reasons for working were almost always economic, women today work just as much for fulfilment, to use their education and training, or simply to help combat the new loneliness and loss of identity which seems so much part of urban living.

But the modern woman has yet another role, the sexual role. This again is in striking contrast to her mother and grandmothers, who in the middle-class society in Victorian times were thought far too spiritual and delicate actually to enjoy anything so coarse as sex. In an age when even piano legs were considered improper and had to be covered with frills, it was not surprising that a woman's body should be a secret and a slightly shameful mystery, while sex for a 'nice' woman was something to be endured rather than enjoyed. One British aristocrat was supposed to have observed that during sexual intercourse 'a true lady never moves'.

That story is probably apocryphal, but it does indicate the prevailing attitude. A lady was not expected to be skilled in sex, initiate it, enjoy it, or even be responsive. She was not an equal sexual partner. Today she is. She has been taught to accept and even take some pride in her own sexual nature, and positively conditioned to expect pleasure as well as to give it.

In her middle years, relieved of the fear of pregnancy and the need to 'take precautions', women often experience a new surge of interest in sex. Above all they have a new need for it. With the children gone from home, they often suffer a sense of loss, of not being needed any more, and there can be compensation and comfort in being needed by their sexual partner.

At just the time when this sexual bond can be of special help, the menopause can unfortunately produce both physical and psychological complications. Dr William H. Masters, Director of the Reproductive Biology Foundation in St Louis, Missouri, and famous co-author with Virginia Johnson of *Human Sexual Response* and *Human Sexual Inadequacy*, believes that the psychological pressure of society's attitudes towards the menopause adversely affect women in their sexual response at this time.

He said,

Many women approach the menopausal years with grave concern because they've absorbed a lot of nonsense that goes along with our society's concept of the menopause. You're finished, you're through as a woman – that sort of thing. If women are concerned, if they are fearful, if they feel that they are less than complete individuals as they go through the menopause, then of course these concepts can affect sexual function. Anything that makes one question one's sexual effectiveness can interfere with responsivity.

The point at which sexual activity may decline depends on the information and attitudes of both husband and wife. Given a reasonably healthy male as an interesting and interested partner, there is no reason why effective sexual functions can't continue for women into the seventy- and eighty-year old group. Unfortunately it is widely believed that a post-menopausal woman loses her ability to respond sexually. Of course this is nothing more than a great cultural fallacy.

Some women certainly are reputed to retain sexual interest and drive late into life. Princess Metternich, when asked at what age a woman ceases to be capable of sexual love is supposed to have replied, 'I do not know, I am only sixty-five'. Simone de Beauvoir quotes an old lady of eighty, asked the same question, who also said, 'You will have to ask someone older than I'.

It would be interesting to know if there is any correlation between women who remain sexually active and possession of adrenal glands which maintain high oestrogen levels.

As we have seen, the opposite can be true. The shutdown of the ovaries and very low oestrogen levels can produce an atrophic state of the vagina, which makes intercourse painful or sometimes impossible, with indirect reduction in libido.

Experts on sexual response, such as Masters and Johnson, were aware of this physical hazard of the menopause a quarter of a century ago, and were recommending oestrogen replacement therapy even then. Dr Masters said,

We use topical or systemic oestrogen replacement. Administration of adequate amounts of oestrogen reconstitute the pelvic tissues to a state akin to that of the pre-menopausal years. The vaginal mucosa thickens, the lubricative pattern develops with more facility and earlier in the response cycle. A great deal of vaginal distensibility is returned. The uterus returns to a pattern of regularly recurrent contractions rather than a spasm with orgasm, and there is a significant increase in blood supply to the pelvis, which facilitates the rapidity and degree of the female's response. We generally use the oral form of replacement with natural oestrogen and continue it indefinitely.

The story of Frankie Fullam and her husband illustrates graphically the sort of problems the menopause can bring into the life of an ordinary married couple. Frankie and Bill quite deliberately describe themselves as 'ordinary', middle-class and middle-income. Bill was a POW in Japanese hands during the war, but he made a good recovery and settled down to a modest job in the Civil Service. They had one son, now grown up. Perhaps the thing not quite so ordinary about them is their obvious and unembarrassed love for each other. Probably only the strength of this got them through the first terrible years of the menopause before Frankie found out about Hormone Replacement. She described to me exactly what happened.

My periods began to get less in 1965 when I was only forty-five and I began to get awful headaches for which my doctor gave me painkillers. By September 1966, my periods had stopped and I remember my first thought was how lovely to be able to have intercourse without precautions at last. But by Christmas my headaches were terrible and I began to have dizzy spells and blackouts. I went back to my GP in the New Year, and when I told him the periods had stopped he confirmed it was the 'change of life' and 'all quite natural'. He gave me stronger tablets but I felt no better, and had to give up my part-time job as I just couldn't concentrate. I was also getting palpitations which scared me.

The headaches were so severe that my own doctor finally sent me to hospital for tests and X-rays. Again I was told it was just 'the change' and nothing was wrong with me.

As the months went by I started hot flushes and awful vaginal irritation. I was given cream and pain killers but by now I was spending days in bed, feeling really ill, and my husband had to lose time off work to look after me. When I did get up, I would look at myself in the mirror and see an old woman, with dry grey-looking skin. It was not a bit like me, and I really felt like doing away with myself. If I had not had such a good husband, I would have done.

As the years went by I experienced night sweats so severe I had to get up many times during the night and dry myself down. My husband and son by then had got used to getting their own breakfast and sandwiches. I just couldn't do it for them.

Then intercourse started to become painful and I found myself dreading my husband making love to me. The vagina was dry and unyielding and, sensing I could not respond, Bill didn't bother me. I lost all feeling in the breasts too, so that love-play had no meaning for me.

When my husband asked our GP if I was a sick woman, he said, 'Oh no, she is only going through the menopause. It is all quite natural. It is lucky she is not an invalid as many women are during the change.'

This went on for seven years until, in 1973, Frankie read my series on Hormone Replacement in the *London Evening News*. She took the articles to her doctor, who told her firmly that it was nonsense, that she had enough oestrogen in her body, and hormone pills would only throw the balance out and give side-effects. He said 'the change' could go on for ten years and offered her more drugs.

But by now Frankie and Bill had had enough. They went to a doctor privately who specialized in HRT. Full tests were carried out and Frankie's oestrogen level was found to be more or less nil. He also confirmed that the vagina had shrunk and this was causing the pain during intercourse. He put Frankie on natural oestrogen and told her to come back in six weeks. She told me what happened next.

The only side-effect for me was slight indigestion in the first few days. Within the six weeks my headaches, flushes, night sweats and palpitations had all gone.

I saw the specialist again and he remarked how different I looked. My skin was better, I was less tense, and he renewed the prescription for a further three months.

Well, within that time I was feeling sexy and wanting to go to bed with my husband again. You can imagine the joy for both of us after those dreadful years. My breasts had firmed up, the vagina was moist again and there was no discomfort at all when we made love.

Ever since we have had a wonderful life again. I feel young and attractive, my hair has thickened up and my skin is really good. I have masses of energy and it is wonderful to be so well after so long feeling only half a woman and half alive. I am doing a part-time job once more.

I have no side-effects and no withdrawal bleeding on my regime of one tablet a day for twenty-one days, then a week off. When I had a smear test after a year on this treatment, the young doctor would not believe I was nearly fifty-five. My oestrogen level was pre-menopausal. What staggers me is that my own GP, who admits that I look marvellous and that the treatment has done wonders for me, will still not use it for his other patients.

Bill Fullam gave me an interesting view of the husband's bewilderment and misery when severe menopausal problems beset a marriage.

It is terribly puzzling for a man and difficult to know what to do for the best. Frankie used to get in the most awful moods, and would shout at me for no reason at all. She knew she was behaving badly but couldn't stop herself.

I spent days at home because she was too ill to get out of bed and scared to be on her own. I tried humouring her and I tried being firm, telling her to get a grip on herself. To be fair, she tried, but the next bout of headaches and hot flushes would be even worse. I found making her suppress her feelings aggravated things, and decided her tantrums and tears were a safety valve.

We kept thinking it would be over soon and that life would become tranquil and just right between us again, but instead it got worse. She'd be drenched in sweat at night and the doctor just kept on giving her tranquillizers and pain killers. When the vaginal trouble started I more or less stopped trying to make love to her.

That was the position for seven years until she went on oestrogen therapy. Since she was put on oestrogen, she has become cheerful and full of energy, and our love-life is better than it has ever been. But she is also serene and happy and there are no more arguments. In fact Frankie now is the woman I first married.

Frankie had a comparatively early menopause starting at forty-five, but for some women it can come even earlier, either naturally or as a result of surgical removal of the ovaries.

Joan Coady, an attractive and vivacious American woman living just outside New York, told me she began 'the change' when only twenty-eight. She explained,

I became very depressed and my menstrual cycle was irregular. I put on weight, couldn't sleep and didn't want to meet people, to the point of becoming a recluse.

None of this was a bit like me and I lost all interest in sex, which wasn't like me either. I dragged from doctor to doctor, without getting any real help, then I happened to read Dr Wilson's book *Feminine For Ever*, and realized it could be a very early menopause. I went to a doctor who specialized in oestrogen therapy, and he confirmed I had an ovarian deficiency which had caused my low oestrogen level and early change of life. He prescribed natural oestrogen and I've never looked back. I am thirty-seven now and my children fourteen and fifteen. There just aren't enough hours in the day for all I want to do. The whole family has reaped the benefit of the therapy and of my feeling so well again. Certainly our sex life is better than ever.

The complete change in personality and the effect of this on the family was emphasized in another letter from a woman who had her ovaries removed. She wrote,

I changed completely after the operation. I am not the same person. I used to be fun to live with, now I know I must be hell. I feel I have driven my children away from home and I can't blame them. When I complained to my doctor, he simply said, 'After what you had done, you can't expect to be the same'.

An early natural or surgical menopause is a very strong and direct indication for HRT. As one British gynaecologist put it, 'The earlier the menopause the more prolonged and acute the changes and this can put a great strain upon a marriage if replacement therapy is not given.'

So many letters make clear how concerned women are for their families. A British woman wrote,

I am forty-seven and just starting the menopause. I am finding life grim with migraine, palpitations and night sweats. My doctor only gives me pain killers, and the depression and apathy I feel are affecting both my marriage and my job. My poor husband has reached the stage when he waits for me to speak first in case he upsets me in some way. I get very aggressive towards him. My job, which carries a great deal of responsibility, is also suffering. I have difficulty in applying my mind and making decisions.

Another British woman wrote,

Since my ovaries were destroyed by radium some six years ago, I have fluctuated in moods right down to absolute depression. This coupled with migraine, and arthritis in hips and knees (none of which I had ever experienced before) had all combined to reduce me from a basically light-hearted extrovert to a near-neurotic. The thing that worries me most is the effect on the family. It is changing the whole atmosphere of our home. I did suggest to my GP that hormone deficiency might be a contributory factor, but was told he wouldn't give me anything that might 'hold up the change'.

Both these women were intelligent and determined, but neither of them could persuade their own doctor to put them on HRT. In the end both had to change to doctors who prescribed Hormone Replacement Therapy, which in both cases proved a complete answer.

Time and again women have emphasized the effect of their own menopause problems on their adolescent children, with minor mutinies blown up into something far more serious by their mishandling or over-dramatizing the situation. One mother wrote,

I can see now that it was my irrational behaviour which finally drove our daughter away from home. My mixture of tears and tantrums made her life a misery. Now, after only a few months on oestrogen, I am my old self again with the hot flushes, depression and exhaustion all gone, but the damage is done. If only I had known about HRT before so that the unnecessary rows and premature breakup of the family could have been avoided.

One concerned daughter actually wrote to me herself putting the family problem. She stated,

My mother is forty-seven and has had all the menopause symptoms described, for the last two years. She is very 'touchy' and yet the next minute can be in floods of tears. When she consulted her doctor she was fobbed off with 'It is your age', which was not a very comforting attitude. Could you let us have the address of a clinic?

Often it is clear that jobs as well as family suffer. Women in the teaching profession, particularly those in mixed schools, find menopausal flushes embarrassing and menopausal confusion and lack of confidence very detrimental to their work. But it applies in ordinary business life too. One woman wrote,

I have recently turned down a good post because I know that when I flush from the toes upwards and feel like crawling into a corner, I just could not face a large office. So, although I have the ability and could earn a great deal more, I stay in my safe little job and resign myself to that.

Another woman who had always helped her husband in the family business wrote,

Each visit my doctor told me my symptoms were natural at my age. I was then forty-three and he advised me to make one room in my house my private retreat and to spend most of my time there away from the demands of the family. As I help my husband run our business, I didn't seem able to impress on him that I just wanted the strength to live normally. All he gave me was Valium to help me sleep and some tablets for energy which sent me so demented that my husband stopped me taking them. I could no longer drive a car, which had been necessary in our business, and my days were a succession of incompleted tasks. Forgetfulness was now added to the nightmare and I wondered if it was premature senile decay.

After she had been put in touch with a clinic this same woman wrote again,

Only to let you know I have been on HRT for almost two cycles. The change is miraculous both physically and mentally. I can now do a really good day's work. I can plan my life and cope with my problems and feel better than I have felt for years.

So HRT is clearly the answer in many cases where the menopause appears to threaten a woman, her family or her job. Happily the picture painted in so many of these letters is no longer generally true. The situation has improved and continues to do so, with HRT now prescribed under the NHS by the great majority of GPs. However, in just a few areas provision can still be patchy and this will persist if expectations continue to be low, and accurate information on HRT not available.

Women need to know what HRT is and what it can do, so that if they do encounter lingering reluctance or obstruction, they will have the confidence and determination to invoke Patient Power as prescribed in the *Patient's Charter*, and their right to hormone treatment as advocated by leading gynaecologists.

In America I found the situation was very different. Through private, though expensive, medicine, women bought both choice and power. As one explained,

I simply told my doctor, when I knew the menopause was starting, that I wanted to be put on replacement hormones. He was not too keen at first, but I simply told him if he didn't give it to me, I should go elsewhere. I knew a lot of my friends were on it and got it from their doctors. Now my own doctor has become convinced about the benefits, seeing how well it works for me and he prescribes it for other patients.

This sort of successful pressure on the doctor to comply with a patient's wishes is very alien to British medicine and certainly could not operate under the National Health Service. While middle-income American women automatically go to a gynaecologist for all their female problems, the British woman and her family is usually registered under the NHS with a local General Practitioner and only sees a specialist on his recommendation, if something arises which requires special investigation, treatment or surgery.

The final chapter will offer a more detailed comparison of the systems, but apart from any financial advantage to the patient in the British system, there is the advantage of the GP knowing the whole family and the circumstances in which they live, which can be relevant to appropriate medical treatment and decisions.

But the disadvantage is that some GPs can at times be autocratic. They do not always feel they must necessarily comply with their patients' wishes. What is more, with only a small per capita payment under the NHS for each patient registered regardless of the number of consultations, they may also be quite happy to let awkward or demanding menopausal patients go elsewhere quite unregretted.

Where a doctor is not prepared to change his or her views, because this would conflict with some personal deeply held and *informed* professional opinion, this can be justified. Where it is simply a matter of clinging to vague uninformed prejudices it is not.

Today we are urged towards more of a partnership with our GPs, and certainly many of the younger doctors in general practice encourage this, adopting a far less formal approach. All the same, pressure under the British system of socialized medicine, with such busy surgeries and usually limited consultation time, tends to produce a somewhat supine patient, often hesitating to offend the GP who looks after her whole family, and afraid in crowded urban areas to consider changing doctors for fear of the very real problem of finding another to take them on.

It is a measure of the depth of desperation and strength of feeling among women on this issue of Hormone Replacement at the menopause, that so many have been prepared to change doctors if that was the only way of getting the treatment. It is also a measure of the change education has brought about in the attitudes and status of women that so many are no longer prepared to be treated, as one woman put it, 'as mindless idiots who have no right to be told anything and must simply obey their doctors without explanation or question'. Another put it even more succinctly: 'Some doctors seem to feel a woman should only open her mouth to swallow his pills'.

A woman today, faced with a doctor who refuses to consider seriously her request for HRT, should open her mouth loud and long in protest. The appalling osteoporosis figures provide her with the strongest possible argument for treatment. No doctor can refute these, nor justifiably reject the advice of the Royal College of Physicians, which urged GPs to prescribe HRT more widely, to reduce those figures. Nor can they ignore indisputable evidence that HRT also halves the incidence of heart attacks and strokes.

Chapter 9

Oestrogens, ageing and depression

It would be a pity if the criticisms made in this book of some doctors' attitudes towards their patients and towards their menopause problems should suggest any bias on my part against the profession in general. On the contrary, in the years researching and writing on medical and social problems, I have found doctors to be almost without exception truly concerned for their patients, dedicated to their work, and remarkably long-suffering with a lay journalist seeking knowledge. They are also blessed, and no doubt need to be, with a special and delightful sense of humour, which helps to lighten what must at times be a grim occupation.

One example of this was the wry joke told me by Sir John Peel, the Queen's former gynaecologist, now retired. We were discussing the need for women to come to terms with ageing, when he suddenly popped in the not entirely relevant story of the man who had suffered his first heart attack and asked his doctor what he should do about sex. 'No excitement, old man,' the doctor replied, 'stick to the wife.'

I appreciated that story. I also appreciated Sir John Peel's fair and sane approach to Hormone Replacement Therapy. Here was a man at the very top of his profession, a truly establishment figure, who was still prepared to allow me to quote him on this controversial question. He told me,

I have used natural oestrogen and cyclic combined hormone therapy for patients over quite long periods, for as much as ten years in some cases. There is no doubt it is of immense clinical benefit to some women between the ages of forty-five and fifty-five and does slow down some ageing processes for a time. Generally my patients are prepared to call a halt themselves at around sixty and I prefer this. At that point they are perhaps more ready to accept ageing.

Sir John's reservations about continuing the therapy into old age are rooted in the fact that other ageing processes still go on, and he, therefore, questions the value of the American rationale of 'oestrogen for ever'. Consensus medical opinion today would agree with this, and recommends preferably eight to ten years on HRT for maximum bone protection.

In America in particular, I did meet many women who had been on oestrogen replacement for over twenty years and were still thriving on it well into their seventies and eighties. One of them was Robert Wilson's own wife, Thelma. It is always a good test of a doctor's faith in his own treatment if he uses it on his own family, and this pioneer of HRT was certainly not afraid to prescribe the treatment for his own wife in the very early days when it was still highly controversial medicine. After over twenty years on cyclic HRT, and then seventy-two, Thelma Wilson was healthy, active and looked far younger than her years. She was then still travelling and lecturing widely as well as walking, golfing and painting in her spare time.

Equally striking was Dr Jessica Marmoston, aged seventy-one, whom I met at the University of Southern California County Medical Center. The normal retiring age is sixty-five, but Dr Marmoston still retained her position as Senior Attendant Physician and Clinical Professor of Medicine. She lived in Los Angeles with her famous film-producer husband, Lawrence Weingarten and took a swim in her pool most mornings before setting out for the ten-mile drive to the hospital. She told me,

I have used oestrogen myself since I was forty-five. I have three children, now grown up of course, but I have always led a very busy life. Oestrogen therapy not only eliminates the usual menopausal symptoms, as I've proved personally and in my clinics, but researches in my own Heart Clinic have shown that oestrogens reduce the risk of arteriosclerosis and heart trouble. Oestrogen therapy seems to have some influence on the incidence of cancer in post-menopausal women. Of four hundred such women under treatment in our clinic, one half of them were given oestrogen and the other half were not. Only one incidence of cancer occurred among the oestrogen-treated patients, and that had occurred prior to therapy in an organ which does not respond directly to oestrogen. In contrast, seven cancers occurred in the patients not receiving oestrogen and two died. I still use oestrogen and it continues to give me the energy to cope with long hours. Often when I get home from the hospital there is still a great deal of work to be done in preparation for next day's clinic.[1]

Of course get-up-and-go is very much an American characteristic anyway, but it seemed particularly abundant in women on HRT, even in the older groups.

But in England too, I met a remarkable seventy-three-year-old doctor, who looked twenty years younger than her age, and who had been on oestrogen for well over twenty years. Dr Greta Malmberg told me,

I could see the medical logic of the concept. I had married late to a man nine years younger than myself so had specially good reasons for wanting to keep young. I have been on HRT for many years now and feel absolutely fine. I still lead a busy professional life as well as running my home.

Writing this update so many years after that interview, it's strange to realize that I am older now than Dr Malmberg was then. Writing in my own mid-seventies, I can pay personal tribute to the benefits of long-term HRT. Over twenty years on treatment have not conferred eternal youth, but hopefully I don't look my age and, more importantly, I don't feel it. I still enjoy tennis and surfing, albeit confined to shorter games and smaller waves. That HRT helps older women keep alert and active is constantly reaffirmed by studies in geriatric centres.

Age is not simply a matter of years. It is a subtle interaction between our physical and mental states and the amount of involvement, interest and activity we are able to maintain. American comedian, Jack Benny, was quoted as saying, 'Age is a question of mind over matter. If you don't mind, it doesn't matter', and there is a good deal of truth behind the quip.

It is much easier not to mind the facts of ageing if you feel well enough and energetic enough to continue your interests, maintain independence, retain identity and preserve dignity.

But with or without oestrogen therapy, in the present state of medical knowledge, sooner or later the physical signs of ageing have to be faced.

To the extent that HRT induces a sense of well-being and renewed energy, to the extent that it keeps the vagina young and healthy enabling normal sex life to continue, to the extent that it keeps skin, hair and bone healthy, preserves muscle tone and helps to check middle-aged spread, to this extent the therapy can help to keep a woman young.

Obviously any cosmetic and rejuvenation effects of HRT are of immense importance to women, but advocates are usually careful not to over-stress them or suggest that oestrogen is some magic elixir of youth.

What oestrogen replacement can do is help a woman to age physiologically instead of pathologically. Robert Wilson himself put it to me this way. He said,

We do not claim that cyclic oestrogen therapy rejuvenates or even prevents ageing, but it does slow it down, makes it a more gentle and gracious process, so that the way a woman ages parallels that of a man. There is no abrupt crisis, no total loss of femininity. Without this help, although modern diets, cosmetics and fashion may make a woman outwardly look even younger than her husband, her body still betrays her. She loses her confidence in herself at the very moment when she is free and most able to enjoy her life.

One of the ways in which accelerated ageing after the menopause makes a woman's body betray her is in the effect of oestrogen deficiency on the skin, which becomes dry, papery and wrinkled. It can be a traumatic experience for a woman to look in her mirror in the cold light of day and see these changes. Vast sums of money are spent by women on various cosmetic techniques designed to conceal or rejuvenate. But the result, as one writer puts it, is usually three stages of woman – childhood, youth, and 'you look wonderful'.

'You look wonderful' in this context too often only means, 'You look wonderful for your age and full marks for trying'. But the woman in her fifties who has the time, money and motivation to take care of skin and hair can still only do so much. No amount of massage and make-up, however skilled, can fully camouflage the atrophic changes which take place in the tissues with age. Quite apart from the face itself, they show up relentlessly also on the skin of the neck, the inner arm and the inside of the thigh.

Hormone Replacement Therapy does seem to slow down these changes and the fact that oestrogen encourages a certain amount of sodium and water retention helps to prevent some wrinkling.

These cosmetic effects of HRT vary considerably from woman to woman, but in some they are dramatic. Although Frankie Fullam was involved with the more serious problems of oestrogen deficiency, she found that oestrogen replacement not only solved these but also gave her the added bonus of improving skin and hair and generally making her look younger.

Another woman who described the cosmetic effects

to me in detail was Mrs Elizabeth Vann, a fifty-two-year-old British housewife who had been on the therapy nearly three years. She also had a responsible job in the Civil Service and after she ceased to menstruate she ran into the common syndrome of depression, irritability and lack of confidence, all of which affected not only her home life but her job. She also told me she had begun to put on weight round the hips and thighs, her breasts had shrunk and her hair was lifeless and thinning.

Mrs Vann was put on natural oestrogen with cyclic progesterone. She told me,

My figure slimmed off again and my breasts improved. It sounds rather immodest but really HRT has done wonders for me. My hair is thick and glossy again and my skin marvellous. In particular that crêpey chicken look I was getting round the neck has disappeared. My legs, which were flabby, have firmed up and my hands, which had never been very good, have at least lost the wrinkly veiny look. When I was out with my sister recently, who is six years younger than I am, I was taken for her daughter.

Although there is plenty of this sort of testimony and doctors too have noted from observation of patients that HRT usually improves elasticity and tone of the skin, there have not been many actual scientific studies done. But at the International Health Foundation Workshop held in Geneva in 1972, Finnish gynaecologists, Professors Rauramo and Punnonen, reported experiments with three separate groups of fifty women, all of whom had had ovaries removed. In each case before the operation a piece of skin was taken from the thigh for biopsy, and thickness and rate of mitosis (cell division) measured.

A month after the operation, two of the groups were put each on a different oestrogen, while the third group went untreated.

At three months and again at six months, more skin

was removed from a place adjacent to the first piece and further biopsy done. In the untreated women there was significant thinning of the epidermis and decrease in the rate of mitosis. In both groups of treated women there was actual thickening of the epidermis, no decrease in mitosis and clear indications that tissue changes were being prevented.[2]

The effect of oestrogen loss on skin is now known to be related to collagen loss. Collagen, which is part of the framework of bone, also forms a supportive network for skin. After the menopause, just as calcium is lost from the bone, collagen is lost from the skin so that it begins to sag and wrinkle. Loss of oestrogen, as we have seen, can also result in very dry and flaky skin. Restoring oestrogen helps to slow down the process, and one recent study at a London Hospital showed skin quality was very much better maintained on HRT, with treated women having thicker, less transparent skin, and fewer lines.[3]

The other way in which the body betrays the post-menopausal woman, affecting health as well as mere vanity, is in weight increase and distribution.

Body weight on average in women increases 12 per cent between the age of twenty and sixty-five, then generally maintains a fairly constant level until the age of eighty when it begins to decrease again.

As with so many symptoms during the menopause, it is difficult to know just how much 'middle-aged spread' is due directly to changing habits and related ageing processes.

Older women do tend to take less exercise and are less active, which means less food is burned up as energy though they usually continue to eat just as much. In fact in some cases the joys of eating seem to become a form of compensation for other things they feel they are missing, and so food intake actually increases. This happens particularly with women who are bored and lonely, or who have perhaps become tired and discouraged by the obvious signs of ageing they perceive in themselves. One way or another it can add up to lack of motivation to restrict their diet or to try to preserve their figure.

Reporting for earlier editions, I was only able to quote one controlled study on weight increase in relation to HRT. Dr Lauritzen, a gynaecologist at the University of Ulm, has published a paper describing how he followed a group of 136 patients treated with natural oestrogen over a period of three years, and compared their weight increase in that time against a control group of untreated patients of the same age. He found weight increases to be significantly greater in the non-treated group.[4]

In the mid-1990s far more studies are available which look at weight gain around the time of menopause, and at how or *if* it is affected by use of HRT.

Despite perceptions by women that HRT (and the Pill) can both cause weight gain, very little evidence for this emerges,[5] though the fluid retention some women experience on oestrogen can give this impression. Results strongly suggest, however, that rather than engendering weight gain, the menopause often serves simply to raise awareness of the *age*-related body changes that are gradually taking place and which, as mentioned, often include weight gain.

One population study of 1496 women aged fifty-five to seventy-four actually found those on oestrogen were slimmer than non-users across all age groups,[6] and again in 1990 a US study involving 40,980 women aged fifty-five to sixty-nine found those who had ever used HRT to have a significantly lower body mass index than those who had never used it.[7]

In Britain the Twin Research Unit, at St Thomas's Hospital, London, reported in *New Scientist* magazine in 1996 that a study involving 560 women found those taking HRT had less body fat overall, and in particular 9 per cent less fat around their abdomens.

A helpful overview of twenty-four such papers published by the International Health Foundation came to the conclusion that any weight gain on HRT is more likely to be related to age-dependent factors than hormonal influence, with a change of lifestyle more effective in reducing weight than just stopping treatment.

Where other ageing changes are concerned, in early research at the University of Tokyo, Dr Hajimo Orimo showed that administration of oestrogen could prevent or delay onset of many of these in female rats![8]

It is a big jump from rats to humans, but ageing today is seen as originating at the cellular level in a process common to all species. Unlike rats, however, women are conscious of their own ageing and the abrupt atrophic changes that follow menopause can often cause distress in our youth-orientated society.

Deterioration in the hair, nails, skin and figure, however, even if accepted by doctors as related to oestrogen deficiency, are unlikely to be considered medically important, at least compared to serious effects of the menopause such as osteoporosis. And there is a curiously puritanical school of thought in medicine which questions the ethics of prescribing HRT simply to increase energy and well-being or to slow down ageing. These physicians question the right of any woman to receive treatment, unless she also displays classic menopause symptoms, or falls into a high-risk category for osteoporosis or heart disease.

Such attitudes are not only held by some elderly family doctors, who can be better forgiven for an old-fashioned medical and social stance, but with far less excuse by younger gynaecologists. Some women who have come up against this sort of attitude feel that occasionally it is rooted, albeit subconsciously, in male determination to keep the one biological advantage they have always had – their ability to age more slowly and retain sexual vigour longer.

Within the British National Health Service, where

finance and facilities are limited and priorities compete and clash, it could be difficult to sustain a strong argument for HRT if it was wanted purely for cosmetic reasons.

But on a private and paying basis, if a woman wants HRT largely, or even only, because she feels it may help her to stay younger longer, then she surely has the right to buy it. If she is prepared to pay for the consultations, test and yearly or twice-yearly follow-up, as well as her regular supply of oestrogen, this is her choice. And it is by no means the choice and prerogative only of rich women, for in relative terms HRT is not an expensive procedure. It is comparable to the cost of the contraceptive Pill, and a woman may well prefer to spend £2 a week on a supply of oestrogen rather than on cigarettes. There is no doubt which will do her more good.

In this connection there was a certain irony in my conversation with one young doctor. I had been invited to talk to a British medical society about Hormone Replacement Therapy. As we stood around afterwards discussing the pros and cons, one GP insisted strongly, 'I feel I should only prescribe oestrogen when it is absolutely necessary, and then for as short a time as possible. After all, the long-term effects are still not really known'. As he spoke he was puffing away at a cigarette, apparently unconcerned about the *known* long-term effects of this drug on himself, or about the fact that he was forcing others to share the proven risk of lung cancer by polluting the air we all breathed.

Disentangling symptoms directly due to the menopause from problems arising out of ageing and out of the normal stresses of life in the mid-years is always difficult. The truth is that both persist alongside each other in a sort of mutual aggravation. The already stressed situation makes menopausal problems worse, and the menopausal symptoms superimposed on the others often add up to a situation in which a woman carries a double load of depression, irritability, fatigue and insomnia.

Work done by Dr Jaszmann, a gynaecologist from Holland, was particularly revealing about these psychosomatic symptoms, previously dismissed by many doctors as not properly belonging to the menopause at all. Dr Jaszmann had the cooperation of some 6000 women all from one urbanized rural community and all between forty and sixty years. He divided them into biological age groups, according to how long it was since their final menstrual period. Then with their help he analysed and plotted as graphs the percentage of the women in each biological age group suffering from each symptom. The result was a series of lines peaking at certain times following final menstruation. For example, hot flushes, pains in muscles and joints, formication and night sweats were all most frequently reported by women in the early post-menopause, and so the line for each of these symptoms peaked at a point within three years of ceasing to menstruate.

The psychosomatic symptoms, fatigue, headaches, irritability, dizziness and depression peaked much earlier when menstruation was starting to become irregular. Breathlessness, palpitations and actual mental unbalance did not show a real peak at all in any biological age group, and from this Dr Jaszmann concluded these symptoms were not truly menopausal. Sleeplessness showed a special pattern peaking five years after final menstruation but continuing high, so that it seemed to be a geriatric complaint rather than a solely post-menopausal one.[9]

The first real scientific evidence that depression can on occasions be linked with oestrogen deficiency came out of a series of double-blind trials carried out in the 1970s at the Merthyr Tydfil General Hospital, Glamorgan.

The Hamilton Depression Scale was used to score the severity of symptoms, oestrogen levels were established by vaginal cytology, and blood tests were also done to establish the level of free tryptophan (an amino-acid) in the blood. This biochemical aspect of the experiment was important, because previous work done by Dr Aylward and his team had shown that concentrations of free tryptophan in the blood were significantly lower in menopausal depressive patients than in corresponding controls. It had also established that certain natural oestrogens could increase the level of free tryptophan.

So a group of women were chosen who had had ovaries removed and who showed depression in addition to the usual accepted features of oestrogen deficiency. Initial blood tests established that the levels of free plasma tryptophan were significantly lower in this study group than in a control group of women of similar age-range and socio-economic status who were not depressive.

But after treatment for three months with an oestrogen (Harmogen) amounts of free plasma tryptophan in the study group were found to have increased to a point at which there was no significant difference in levels between them and the control group. What is more, these same patients showed an improvement in depression, with scores which correlated with the increase in free tryptophan.

This research was particularly important not only because it was the first to show that depression can be directly linked to lack of oestrogen, but because it also indicated how the oestrogen–depression link may work through the influence of oestrogen in raising free plasma tryptophan levels. Finally, of course, it showed the adminstered oestrogen can also raise the tryptophan level and improve the depression.[10]

Over the years other studies have further confirmed the value of HRT in relieving menopausal depression. And where oestrogen has been prescribed for physical menopause problems, its ability also to relieve associated depression has been repeatedly demonstrated in clinical practice. Despite this, where women present with depression only, in the *absence* of other physical menopause symptoms, doctors still tend to prescribe tranquillizers or antidepressants.

In April 1996, however, *The Lancet* carried details of work which confirmed oestrogen to be highly effective in treating another form of female depression. Doctors in London and Salisbury studied a group of over sixty women, all suffering from post-natal depression, a condition often lasting six to twelve months and notoriously unresponsive to tranquillizers or antidepressants.

Some of the women were allocated oestrogen skin patches to wear and others given only dummy patches, with none knowing which kind they were on.

At the end of just one month, women on the active oestrogen showed rapid improvement, fully sustained over the next five months. No similar improvement was found in the placebo group. Apart from obviously concluding that oestrogen patches are likely to prove valuable in treatment of post-natal depression, doctors also felt these findings suggest that, where women are concerned, oestrogen may be equally effective in relieving depression in general.

John Studd, the gynaecologist who led the London team involved in this study, and who is a leading pioneer of HRT in Britain, told me, 'Hopefully this may help to convince doctors of the hormonal nature of much of the depression experienced by women. I've been using oestrogen implants successfully for many years to treat various forms of female depression including that linked to the menopause and to PMS. With the patch both simple and available, hopefully GPs will now at least try oestrogen *before* resorting to antidepressants and tranquillizers so alien to the human body and so liable to turn the patient into a zombie.'

It is accepted, of course, that depression is more common following a surgical menopause than a normal one, and an interesting study confirming this was reported in *The Lancet*, in August, 1973. Dr D. H.

Richards gave the results of a follow-up on 200 patients from his mostly urban group practice near Oxford, all of whom had had hysterectomies. Some sixty-five women had also had both ovaries removed and twelve others had had one removed.

The 200 patients were matched for age and as closely as possible for marital status, etc., against 200 female control patients, who had *not* had the operation.

Depression was defined for the purpose of the study as a condition which when diagnosed by any of the four partners in the practice, was treated with antidepressive drugs.

For 151 women, three years or more had elapsed since their operations, and fifty of them (33 per cent) had had depression within the three years, compared to only eleven (7 per cent) of the matched controls. What is more, nine of the hysterectomy patients required admission to mental hospital, as compared to only one of the controls.

The study showed depression after hysterectomy not only to be four times more frequent, but also more severe and of longer duration, lasting an average 24.6 months as against only 10.9 months in the control group. Almost half of the women developing depression after the operation did so within six months.[11]

Dr Richards's own comments are interesting. He wrote,

The effect of hysterectomy seems in some respects to resemble that of the menopause, but in an exaggerated form. This view is further supported by the study of other signs and symptoms that are characteristic of women who have undergone hysterectomy. It is not uncommon for women who have had hysterectomy to suffer from hot flushes which begin shortly after their operation, irrespective of whether the ovaries have or have not been removed.

This and other symptoms raise the possibility that an endocrine factor may be involved even when the uterus alone is removed. Prospective studies are in progress to establish the degree and nature of endocrine change.

Today there is a considerable body of work confirming Dr Richards's observations, and it is now accepted that hysterectomy in women under forty-five, even where ovaries are conserved, can result in premature menopause occurring in 50 per cent of such cases within four years of surgery.[12] Younger women, those under forty-two years of age at the time of surgery, appear to undergo ovarian failure even earlier, often experiencing hot flushes and sweating within six months.[13] Unless this early onset of the climacteric is recognized and appropriate oestrogen replacement started, such patients will run associated higher risks of osteoporosis and cardio-vascular disease,[14] as well as the increased risk of depression.

It would appear from this that removal of the target organ, the uterus, may discourage the ovaries so that output is reduced and oestrogen levels drop. Or more prosaically the surgery itself may simply have reduced blood supplies to the ovaries, lowering their efficiency.[15]

Whatever the reason may prove to be, if and when a hysterectomy does result in sluggish ovarian function, then obviously HRT is indicated. It is even more firmly indicated, of course, where the hysterectomy is accompanied by removal of both ovaries, producing a surgical menopause that often involves severe oestrogen deficiency symptoms.[16]

Better understanding and greater usage of Hormone Replacement, together with refinements in methods of assessing hormone levels, both contribute today to more and more use of hormonal management actually to avoid the need for some hysterectomies.

Obviously where the symptoms, such as excessive bleeding or discharge, are due to uterine disease, or where there are large fibroids, there is no alternative to surgery. In other cases, where the underlying cause is faulty hormonal balance, then attempts should be made to correct this before the easier resort to the knife. There is some evidence that knife-happy surgeons too often remove symptoms by removing the uterus, without properly establishing the cause and considering alternatives. Critics insist that this is not only an easy way of avoiding time and trouble, but also an easy way of making money. But the opposing argument insists that the uterus serves no purpose other than to carry a baby for nine months, so that once the family is complete, if it is giving trouble it may as well be removed not only to overcome the present problems but to prevent future ones.

It is an appealing argument for the doctor, not quite so appealing for the woman who has to face the discomfort of the surgery and who rightly or wrongly resents losing an important part of her body that carried and nourished her children.

The answer has to be one based on medical knowledge and medical judgement, not on the patient's emotional reaction, but she is entitled to be sure that both judgement and knowledge are used on her behalf. Now it has been established that even simple hysterectomies can have a kick-back effect on the efficient working of the ovaries, there is even more reason for the pros and cons to be properly weighed up.

A letter stressing the effects of the loss of ovaries was sent to me by Joan Bates, a vicar's wife, then living in Somerset. She wrote,

At the age of twenty-nine after only four years of marriage, I had to have both ovaries removed. We were very naive and went ahead at once to adopt a child. But after only six months I collapsed into severe depression. I loved my husband dearly, but experienced such a personality change that I told him to go away. I did not want to be his wife and I lost interest in him, my home, and life itself.

My local GP called in a psychiatrist and I was six months in a Psychiatric Unit, until, in despair, I left, with my husband being told there was 'nothing they could do'.

My husband refused to give up and quite by chance a

friend told him of an endocrinologist. At St Thomas's
Hospital in London I was put on hormone replacement with
artificially induced menstruation. It has been miraculous
and given us back a normal and happy married life. Over
the years we have adopted three children, but I am
convinced I could still be in a psychiatric hospital and on
tranquillizers if it had not been for having a husband
prepared to fight to get me HRT. I am sure there are many
women in such hospitals today being given the wrong
treatment, when their depression like mine may be
hormone-based.

It is largely because of the symptoms of the menopause appear at different biological ages, as Dr
Jaszmann's work so clearly showed, that medicine has
often failed to recognize them for what they are.

To some extent all tissues in the human body can be
regarded as target organs for oestrogens, and the whole
organism, therefore, reacts to oestrogen deficiency in
varying degrees and at varying times. The hypothalmic
centres are affected quickly so that hot flushes come
early in the pattern, whereas bone tissues take a long
time to be affected and so osteoporosis develops late.

This time-lag in the emergence of these symptoms,
and the mixture of physical and psychic complaints,
have confused diagnosis and blurred the picture so that
doctors have recognized only part of it. In particular
they have relied on tranquillizers to curb nervous
effects, instead of oestrogens to eradicate them.

For a time in Great Britain, a sort of half-way house
emerged in HRT prescribing, with some doctors grudg-
ingly accepting the value of the therapy, but only for
short periods, and only to combat clear physical symptoms, such as hot flushes and sweats. If, as a byproduct,
some of the psychosomatic symptoms were also
relieved, there was a tendency to take this as proof that
they were 'all in the mind', rather than accepting
that these too can have a hormone-trigger effect.

What any form of short-term therapy does not take
into account is that when it is stopped, the uncomfort-

able symptoms usually return, and even if they don't, other slow hidden degenerative processes associated with oestrogen deficiency go on.

So let us look at the ways in which Hormone Replacement Therapy is more properly used, and at the practical details of the tests, treatment and choices that face a woman and her doctor.

Chapter 10

The test and the treatment

A changing menstrual pattern is usually a pretty firm indication that oestrogen levels are dropping. For many doctors this signal alone, or taken in conjunction with other menopause symptoms, is enough to allow replacement therapy to be started.

In the US doctors often like to use a simple test actually to establish oestrogen levels. This not only provides a diagnostic confirmation but gives some indication of the oestrogen replacement dosage needed. Later on, when the test is repeated, it also serves to confirm that the replacement therapy is working satisfactorily.

The principle is simple. One of the main functions of oestrogen is to mature the cells of the vagina and keep it healthy and supple. A vaginal smear viewed under the microscope quickly reveals to the practised eye the number of mature cells, compared to the number of intermediate cells and immature cells. This ratio forms what is called the Maturation Index.

Hundreds of tests have already established that the Maturation Index for a normal, healthy, menstruating woman is the area of eighty-five mature cells to fifteen intermediate with no immature cells. This figure varies slightly from woman to woman, and for some it may be nearer seventy-five mature to twenty-five intermediate, but there should be few or no immature cells so long as oestrogen levels are reasonably high.

For the untreated post-menopausal women, however, the index can be completely reversed, so that there are no mature cells and the majority are intermediate or immature. A short time on oestrogen replacement usually brings the index back within the normal range, and this is a strong indication that the therapy is working correctly.

It is important, however, to emphasize that vaginal smears do not always correlate completely with menopause symptoms or with the patient's response to hormone therapy. This is because the smear can be influenced by many other factors, such as *when* it was taken, *where* it was taken from in the vagina, and the presence of vaginal infection such as monilia (thrush). Bleeding, recent intercourse and even the taking of other drugs can also affect the smear, while there is the additional problem of variation in the response of ageing tissues. Biochemical assay methods may reveal quite high levels of oestrogen in the blood, while response of the cells of the vagina may be poor and only give a low Maturation Index.

Another variable to further confuse the issue is the different interpretation of smears by different technicians, when slides have to be sent away to outside laboratories.

It is small wonder that in his excellent book, *The Ageless Woman*, gynaecologist, Sherwin Kaufman, insists, 'Smears are not a dependable measure of the absolute level of oestrogen in the body, especially when a single test is made'. Dr Kaufman goes on to deplore a woman asking to have their 'oestrogen level' checked as though it were oil for an engine, and the female tendency to confuse oestrogen levels with sex appeal. For these reasons, and because today measuring hormone levels in the blood is more simple and accurate, the Maturation Index is rarely used in this country.

Where there is any doubt about the onset of menopause or a patient's hormonal status, British doctors prefer to use modern assay methods, establishing from simple blood tests either the level of oestrogen itself or of follicle-stimulating hormone (FSH). The latter, as the name implies, is concerned with stimulating and ripening eggs, so that once ovaries begin to fail the body responds by producing extra amounts of FSH to try to prod them back into action again. Any rise in this hormone, therefore, means that the symptoms are truly menopausal.

Although a woman in her thirties may present with all the usual symptoms, GPs can still be reluctant to accept this as evidence of true menopause. Yet records show at least 1 per cent of women run into premature menopause – officially designated as the end of menstruation occurring under the age of forty.

The point is, however, that some symptoms, in particular those often termed psychosomatic, such as depression, confusion, irritability and lethargy, can show up well before hormone levels fall sufficiently to bring an end to periods and meet the accepted medical criterion for menopause.

So, if his patient being young blinds a doctor to the true situation, so that the correct diagnosis is not made and HRT not given promptly, repeated studies, as mentioned, have shown that the extra years without circulating oestrogen can result in four times the normal risk of osteoporosis, heart disease and depression. For this reason it is important that any woman who suspects early onset should consult her GP, and, if necessary, insist on a blood test. A hormone assay is not an expensive procedure and can give a definitive answer within a few days.

Jean Simpson, a nurse herself, told me how difficult it had been at only thirty-five to convince her doctor she was menopausal.

My GP simply refused to believe me when I told him my life was being made a misery by hot flushes. Menstruation with me had always been irregular so that he took no notice of this other symptom. I was also very depressed, but again this can happen for other reasons though it had never happened to me previously. I also suffered bone and joint pains which I had never had before. In the end I persuaded him to refer me to a menopause clinic and the hormone levels they found confirmed my ovaries were not working. HRT was explained to me and I was warned that I must be prepared to accept a regular bleed on this treatment. This didn't worry me very much as I had never fully stopped periods and at least on HRT they were light and regular. Flushes disappeared within a week and I began to feel my old self again very quickly. They had explained to me at the clinic that HRT would also prevent the additional bone loss which comes with the menopause. In my case starting the change so young, if it wasn't checked there were a lot of extra years in which my bones could become dangerously brittle. So, the monthly bleed seemed a small price to pay for so many advantages.

One price the HRT monthly bleed does exact for women who start their treatment as Jean did, before final menstruation has occurred, is difficulty in knowing when it is safe to stop using contraception. Their natural menopause onset is, of course, masked by the regular withdrawal bleeds, so the problem is: how can their GP determine if it is yet safe for them to have unprotected intercourse?

Again the FSH test provides useful guidelines. If the blood test shows FSH raised, the crucial menopause moment is not far away. Over fifty this means that barrier methods need be used only for a further six months. If under that age they must be continued for at least eighteen months. In both cases, of course, HRT goes on.

If, however, FSH tests shows *normal* levels, HRT should be stopped for twelve days to allow hormones from it to clear, then another FSH must be done. If that too is normal HRT is re-started and barrier methods must be used, with the whole process being repeated again after another twelve months.

If, however, the second FSH test shows *raised* levels, then barrier methods must again be used but only for six months, with no need for further tests.

All this is not nearly so complicated as it may sound, and avoids loss of HRT protection over the much longer time it could otherwise take to see if natural periods are still taking place, as well as avoiding a late or unwanted pregnancy.

Individual attitudes towards the renewed menstruation that traditional HRT imposes to protect the womb vary considerably. In America I met some women who accepted it happily as keeping them 'female and functioning'! Others would ask to be put on sub-bleeding doses of oestrogen or be stabilized on a longer cycle with a bleed only every two months or every forty-two days. This was quite common especially among older women. Bleeding occurred during the week they were off treatment and in general terms, I found a woman who went on HRT right at the onset of the menopause, or even very soon after her final menstrual period, was more willing to accept continuation or renewal of a monthly bleed than one who may have had a gap of several years since her periods ended. Once out of the habit of bothering with sanitary towels etc, there can be a natural reluctance to start all over again.

One marvellous woman of seventy-plus, who had willingly accepted menstruation for years for the sake of feeling well and keeping young, confided that she had eventually become embarrassed about buying sanitary towels at her age. She told me, 'I pretend now that they are for my daughter, and I vary the stores I buy them from. I really think I may ask my doctor to change the therapy, because I know it is possible to have oestrogen without bleeding'.

This is true, but important British research by Dr Malcolm Whitehead at King's College Hospital showed this absence of bleeding did not necessarily guarantee that there was no gradual build-up of womb lining. Because of this it seems few British doctors are likely to favour prescribing oestrogen alone, even in sub-bleeding doses. If it is ever done in this country, then any good doctor will insist it is only for a few weeks.

Generally, today, medical opinion on HRT round the world tends to favour the lowest dosage of oestrogen to relieve patients' problems and protect their bones. It is also accepted that oestrogen may be prescribed on a *continuous* basis, always providing a twelve-day progestogen course is interposed regularly alongside the oestrogen, ensuring the regular shedding of any build-up of womb lining exactly as in the natural cycle.

From the first, Sir John Peel had advocated the combined therapy. He insisted:

No one should use oestrogen alone and without interruption day in and day out. Prolonged and continuous over-stimulation of the endometrium can be a factor in producing endometrial cancer. I believe the combination with a progestogen is a safer system.

Pharmaceutical companies, who have a strong vested interest in product safety as well as effectiveness, responded to the clear guidelines established by British research with a whole range of 'combined' HRT packs, containing built-in progestogen courses. Prempak and Cycloprogynova led the way, followed by Prempak C, Trisequens, Nuvelle, Climagest and Femoston.

Experience in Britain has shown that where the importance of progestogen to safeguard the womb is properly explained, the need to bleed is accepted. I found here too a few women who welcomed this continuation of a familar cyclical life-rhythm. One British woman told me: 'I think of my body as a machine which needs servicing; HRT is part of that servicing and it keeps my body working properly and, as it were, firing on all cylinders.'

The reaction of fifty-two-year-old Mrs Vann, whose case history was recounted earlier, was equally positive: 'It's not a question of putting up with it,' she said. 'I actually welcome it. It makes me feel young and normal.' However, what may feel normal in a woman's fifties may feel absurd in her seventies, and as they grow older many women choose to come off treatment *unless* there is a strong reason to continue, such as existing osteoporosis or high risk of developing either that or heart disease.

For older women staying on HRT, it may be comforting to know that with age, as the tissues become less responsive to hormone influence, the withdrawal bleed tends to get lighter. Also, of course, a year into the post-menopause, there is now the useful option of switching to one of the *non-bleed* HRT methods described fully later in this chapter.

For women who have had a surgical menopause, of course, the 'to bleed or not to bleed' dilemma does not arise. Without a uterus there is no such complication, and oestrogen alone usually produces excellent results. As one doctor put it to me: 'These women have the best of both worlds, all the advantages of HRT at a proper protective dosage, and no complications with bleeding.'

For others, it is possible to give HRT in doses too low to produce a bleed, but British experts believe they are also too low to properly protect bone and heart. However, other non-bleed forms of HRT have now won unqualified approval in this country for both prompt relief of menopause symptoms and for long-term protection. These are described below together with other new systems now widely used.

Non-bleed systems of HRT
Continuous Combined HRT (CCT) Kliofem and Premique are brand names for the first specially formulated packs providing Continuous Combined HRT (CCT), sometimes known as Non-Sequential HRT.

Both names reflect the fact that instead of the progestogen being given in sequence with oestrogen and confined to the end of the cycle, it is given continuously *alongside* oestrogen every day but with only tiny doses of each hormone used. With this method, there is no build-up of womb lining and so nothing to be shed. However, this no-bleed bonus only holds good if there is little or no natural oestrogen from the ovaries still around. To ensure this it is not recommended for use until a year past final menstruation. Even if this advice is observed, just a few women do experience a little spotting or an occasional bleed during the first six months on this continuous combined system. Their doctors, of course, should always warn them of this possible side-effect and reassure them that it does not usually persist after that initial period. If it does, some other form of HRT should be considered.

Many women settle happily on this treatment, gaining good relief of symptoms and excellent bone protection. In fact, some studies have shown figures for the preservation of bone mass in spine and forearm to be *superior* to those achieved by conventional HRT.

This treatment has been used successfully on the continent for a long time, and even before the general licence was granted here or special packs became available, some British doctors were already prescribing it on a named patient basis, making up their own formulations of daily low doses of a natural oestrogen and progestogen. But although there is good practical experience to back this system, monitoring still continues to evaluate in particular long-term cardiovascular protection.

Livial This non-bleed product, introduced just too late to make the 1990 edition of *No Change*, takes a very innovative approach. It uses a specially developed steroid (Tibilone), which is not really an oestrogen but mimics the *effects* of oestrogen, together with those of progestogen and the male hormone androgen. The result is a form of HRT which gives good relief of symptoms *without* stimulating the womb lining, and so without the need to bleed.

It is important to note, however, that this 'bleed-free' bonus again only obtains if the product is used after the ovaries have *completely* shut down. Accordingly, the makers, Organon, do not recommend Livial either for use in the pre-menopause or immediate post-menopause periods, when even low levels of residual oestrogen can be enough to provoke a bleed. Used a year after final menstruation, however, there is usually no problem.

Studies indicate that Livial also offers very good bone protection, and work so far seems to confirm equally good cardio-protective effect. So, women who start out on conventional HRT and find regular shedding difficult to tolerate now have the option of switching to Livial later. In a few cases bleeds may occur briefly just after the switch-over, usually due to residual oestrogen in the system from the earlier traditional HRT. Doctors should warn patients of this possibility and reassure them that the problem will soon clear.

Bleed-free systems such as Livial, Kliofem and Premique now occupy a useful place in the spectrum of HRT prescribing. They have particular value for women who, despite being at high risk of osteoporosis, reject vital HRT because they cannot face withdrawal bleeds for the five to eight years recommended to ensure maximum bone protection. Just knowing that a year into the menopause they can switch to a non-bleed method which will continue to give the necessary protection can make long-term treatment far more acceptable.

A tricky question may arise for some women when planing to switch to Kliofem or Premique. If, as increasingly happens today, they have been put on HRT early to counter the miserable symptoms that often arise *before* menstruation ceases, there is a problem in knowing when they have reached the necessary year beyond the menopause to qualify for CCT or Livial. The time of final menstruation will have been masked by the regular withdrawal bleeds of traditional HRT.

It is much the same question as that which arises

when deciding whether it is safe to abandon contraception. In the past doctors often just took women right off treatment and made them wait to see if natural periods recurred. As already explained, this could often mean a long wait during which symptoms returned and bone and heart protection were lost. Rather better than that was the system of taking the patient off for just the two or three weeks required to allow residual oestrogen from HRT to clear the system, and then doing a blood test to establish oestrogen levels and confirm menopause status.

Today, however, another and more ingenious method has become possible and is being widely used. It was described to me by consultant gynaecologist, Peter Bowen-Simpkin, a leading expert on HRT: 'We switch the patient straight to Livial, which contains no actual oestrogen,' he explained. 'Then for the last twelve days of the cycle we prescribe a progestogen. If a bleed then follows, this indicates some oestrogen is still present and it must have been produced by the body. In that case,' he went on, 'the menopause has *not* occurred and the patient must go back for some time longer to traditional HRT. But if no bleed occurs, then menopause is past and Livial can be continued or Kliofem or Premique used.'

The transdermal patch Another popular newcomer to the HRT scene in the early 1990s has been the transdermal patch, widely prescribed now by GPs and gynaecologists. This consists of a small thin transparent patch which the user attaches to the skin of abdomen or thigh. Natural oestrogen, oestradiol, is then released at a constant rate through the skin direct into the bloodstream. This is physiologically closer to natural ovarian action, avoiding the sudden surge of hormones produced by tablets, and avoiding also loss in the digestive tract, so allowing a lower dose to be effective. It also eliminates the possible digestive upsets that can plague a few women on oral HRT. The patch has proved to give excellent relief of immediate overt symptoms, and at 50 mcg (microgram) strength it also protects bone, heart and arteries.

Estraderm This is the only patch to hold oestrogen in a small reservoir of alcohol, surrounded by adhesive and sandwiched between clear layers of film. The sticky contact layer is perforated by thousands of tiny holes through which the oestrogen is absorbed into the skin. It must be renewed twice a week (every three or four days) and comes in 25-mcg and 50-mcg strengths. The higher dose is necessary for full bone protection.

Evorel This is also a twice-a-week patch. Like all others except Estraderm, it presents the oestrogen actually mixed with the adhesive and spread right across a single layer of clear film. Known as 'matrix'-type patches, these are claimed to provide greater sticking power. Patches certainly can sometimes go adrift, especially in hot humid climates, in the bath, or even occasionally during intercourse. It has been known for a patch to end up adorning the male partner – not a desirable state of affairs, as oestrogen does nothing for the male libido!

Fematrix This later matrix patch, which came onto the market in 1995, also requires changing every three or four days, and comes in 80-mcg strength.

Menorest This is another matrix twice-a-week patch, for which a claim of *no* skin irritation is made.

Progynova TS This matrix patch broke really new ground in 1996 by having to be changed only *once* a week, which it is thought users may find easier to remember. Again it releases natural oestradiol at 50 mcg per day with a stronger (100-mcg) patch also available.

Femseven This other seven-day patch, also coming out in 1996, deserves special mention as the first HRT product to achieve official licence not only for menopause symptoms and osteoporosis, but as stated on the data sheet '*for reduction of the increased risk of cardiovascular events in postmenopausal women with symptomatic coronary artery disease*'.

The same indication will surely now be sought (and logically should be granted) for all other oestrogen patches. One would, indeed, expect it to be given to all other HRT products based on natural oestrogen. Such positive recognition on data sheets of the value of HRT for cardio-vascular protection might at last banish any lingering misconception of heart or artery disease being seen as contra-indications for HRT. Exactly the opposite has been proven and officially accepted, with data sheets and pharmaceutical reference books amended accordingly, though not yet in the same very positive terms.

With all patches, despite makers' claims, just a few women do suffer adverse skin reaction, and it is advisable when renewing to slightly change the position to minimize any risk of contact soreness. If this problem occurs with one type of patch, it is always worth trying a different make before switching to some other form of HRT. With all the many methods and products now available, it's very much a question of horses for courses and of finding the system and preparation that best suits *you*.

All the patches mentioned up to now supply only oestrogen and so are more convenient for women who have had a hysterectomy. Other users with a womb to protect still need to take regular courses of oral progestogen, and special calendar packs have been designed to simplify this.

Evorel-Pak This offers 50-mcg Evorel patches plus twelve tablets of norethisterone supplying the progestogen.

Estrapak 50 This comprises estraderm patches, again with twelve 1-mg tablets of norethisterone.

Femoston This consists of Fematrix patches with twelve days of progestogen included, but this time in the form of Duphaston tablets (dydrogesterone).

Estracombi This is the only truly combined patch, which brilliantly eliminates any need for oral progestogen. Anticipated in the last edition of *No Change*, the combined patch has since been licensed for use and is especially suitable for the many women who have *not* had a hysterectomy. Each pack contains two sets of patches: the first delivers just 50 mcg oestradiol for two weeks; the second set then delivers both oestrogen and progestogen for the last two weeks. Both hormones go directly into the bloodstream, so that a much lower dosage of progestogen can be used than with oral HRT. It is hoped that this lower dose may help women who suffer PMS-type symptoms in the progestogen phrase of their cycle.

Other transdermal methods

Oestrogel This transdermal HRT product is new to the UK though it has long been used in Europe. Presented as a colourless skin gel, it can be rubbed on the forearm or inner thigh, contains the same type of natural oestrogen as in the patch and is equally well absorbed into the skin. However, the area used needs to be kept bare for five minutes and dry for an hour. The gel is contained in a small pump dispenser and the dose is adjustable. Non-hysterectomized women, of course, still need to take a separate progestogen.

Implants Another system designed to deliver oestrogen direct into the bloodstream is the subcutaneous implant. This involves a very minor surgical procedure, but one that few GPs have bothered to master. Implants are usually only available at menopause clinics or from gynaecologists. Chapter 12 describes the method in full detail.

Vaginal oestrogens These are usually prescribed in the form of creams, pessaries or tablets and are most applicable where menopause symptoms are confined to vaginal dryness or urinary problems. Absorption can be irregular and although they are described as 'topical', there can still be systemic effects, with high doses even causing sufficient build-up of womb lining to result in unexpected bleeds. Because of this, some doctors consider that a course of progestogen needs to be taken, although bleeds are very unlikely with low-dose oestradiol vaginal tablets or with oestradiol creams.

One of the creams, Dienostrol, is based on a synthetic oestrogen, and there is no longer any need for doctors to prescribe this when there are alternatives: Ovestin, based on the natural oestrogen, oestriol, or Premarin Cream based on natural conjugated oestrogens.

Tampovagan　Even more to be avoided is this pessary based on synthetic stilbestrol. As already explained this has no place at all in HRT and women should ask instead for Ortho-Gynest pessaries based on natural oestriol.

Vagifem　These vaginal tablets, also based on natural oestrogen, offer another alternative for restricted local treatment.

Many women find creams and pessaries messy, but more importantly they do not offer protection against osteoporosis or cardio-vascular disease. In view of these limitations, it is difficult to feel enthusiastic about them when there are equally safe methods that offer more benefits.

Estring　Another and better vaginal option has become available with the arrival of this oestrogen ring. Soft, slightly flexible and impregnated with oestrogen, this sits towards the top of the vagina so comfortably that the wearer can forget its presence. Fitted by the doctor, it only has to be renewed every three months. During that time low-dose oestrogen is slowly released at a consistent rate, and without the mess or the trouble involved with creams and pessaries. At the moment a week's break is recommended before the next ring is inserted to allow any minor changes in womb lining to regress.

A new form of oral HRT, Tridestra, deserves special mention as it demands a withdrawal bleed only once every three months. This is obviously good news for women who find it difficult to tolerate the bleed every month imposed by other traditional combined HRT tablets. Packs of Tridestra are designed for easy use, with the first 91 white tablets containing only oestrogen and the following 14 blue ones a combination of oestrogen and progestogen; the final 7 yellow tablets have no active ingredient, so that each course ends with a hormone-free week.

The addition of these placebo tablets maintains regular progress through each three-month course, cutting the risk of forgetting to start again after what would otherwise be a blank week. Back in the mid-1970s, early British research established that up to three months on oestrogen alone was safe, always providing it was followed by a course of progestogen, as in this case.

So treatment choice grows wider but, despite all the different types of HRT and the different ways of taking it that are now available, the basic concept and purpose remains the same – the replacement of missing hormones – the remedy of a deficiency state.

Chapter 11

The choice of oestrogens

As well as a choice of techniques and regimens, there is also, of course, a choice of oestrogens. Although so far throughout this book reference has been made to 'oestrogen', as though it were one single substance, in fact there is a whole family of these hormones secreted by the ovaries during their functioning life.

Although it was only at the beginning of this century that the hormonal nature of ovarian control of reproduction was established, and only in the 1920s that female sex hormones themselves were discovered in the urine of menstruating and pregnant women, ancient remedies were often based on placental material which is rich in oestrogen and on urine which also contains sex hormones.

The use of human placenta was first mentioned in a Chinese pharmacopoeia of AD 725, but may go back even further. Certainly by the fourteenth century it was commonly prescribed in China for all forms of debility including sexual weakness. One Chinese doctor of that period wrote,

I have often used it and obtained perfect results, especially in female patients. The merit of the placenta is chiefly to increase the efficiency of the Yin force in the body, including sexual function. It always seems to give good results. If one takes it for a long time it improves the hearing, brightens the eyes, keeps the hair and beard black, increases longevity, and indeed has such merit that it can overcome the natural process of ageing.

Even more remarkable than the unwitting use so long ago of oestrogen from the placenta, was the development of medieval Chinese medicine to include fractionation of urine, yielding end-products which quite certainly included both androgens and oestrogens.

The use of urine in the ancient medicine of many nations was written off in modern times as useless and disgusting, until the classical discovery of S. Ascheim and B. Zondek in 1927 of the presence of large amounts of sex hormones in pregnancy urine, and the subsequent discovery that the urine of all animals, but especially that of the mare, contain these substances. The horse in fact has been described as a remarkable oestrogen factory, and the pregnant mare excretes over 100 mg daily.

Many of the family of naturally occurring oestrogens can be successfully synthesized in the laboratory, sometimes modified slightly in structure by linking with a salt. Examples include piperazine oestrone sulphate (Harmogen) which is proving a useful oestrogen for replacement therapy, and estradiol valerate (Progynova) introduced in the UK in 1975.

A sharp distinction should be made between such manmade versions of naturally occurring oestrogens, and those correctly termed 'synthetic oestrogens', such as stilbestrol and dienoestrol. These are entirely artificial both in chemical and molecular structure, do not occur in nature and are essentially foreign to the human body.

These truly synthetic oestrogens are merely substances which possess oestrogenic-like properties, and many have been developed specifically as the basis of the contraceptive Pill and for its distinctly *unnatural* task of maintaining a permanent state of infertility. For this purpose they are extremely effective.

They do, however, have certain side-effects and hazards, in particular an effect on blood-clotting potential with slightly increased thrombosis risk. With the wide choice of naturally occurring oestrogens now available and where no contraceptive purpose is required, it seems outdated and outmoded to still prescribe synthetic oestrogens for treatment of the menopause.

An exception to this might prove to be the sophisticated sequential concept of a preparation like Menophase, when varied doses of the synthetic oestrogen, Mestranol, are given in a carefully calculated sequence. Over the last thirteen days, the oestrogen is also combined with a progesterone, so that the body's own pre-menopause pattern of rise and fall in sex hormone levels is closely simulated. This was the technique used in the HRT clinic at Birmingham Women's Hospital, with the satisfactory and interesting results already reported.[1]

At one time letters from women and contact with doctors made it clear that other synthetic oestrogens, particularly stilbestrol, were being used far too often to relieve menopause symptoms instead of the safer naturally occurring oestrogens. It was obvious that some family doctors did not even appreciate the distinction between synthetic and naturally occurring oestrogens, and had missed research reports indicating that the latter are free from thrombosis risk.

I hasten to add that it is not difficult to sympathize with over-worked GPs who simply do not have time to keep up with the vast outpourings of medical literature. It is less easy to sympathize with those who huff and puff about there being no such literature on Hormone Replacement. In fact the bibliography at the back of just one booklet sent by one drug company to all doctors lists 114 papers and research sources.

From personal experience I can vouch for familiarity with hundreds more, as the piles of papers stacked on my desk bear witness. The writer of one such paper made a wry comment about doctors who grumble that there is no HRT literature. He said, 'Maybe their definition of literature is what they read, not what is written'.

Natural conjugated oestrogen (Premarin), most commonly used to treat the menopause, even today is refined direct from the urine of pregnant mares. It contains the whole range of oestrogens which the body before the menopause both produces and responds to. This multiple-oestrogen content, is the reason for some doctors' preference, as they believe it should ensure wider application and relief of symptoms.

On the first television programme ever done on Hormone Replacement Therapy in the UK, which I presented for Associated Television's enterprising 'Women Today', the young gynaecologist who had been invited to oppose the concept opened his spirited attack by scoffing at the notion of equine oestrogen as 'natural'. 'Natural to what?' he asked, 'Natural to horses?'

It was a fair enough debating point, and obviously the ideal oestrogen for the ideal replacement therapy would be *human* conjugated oestrogen. In the very early days of the therapy this was even possible, with hormone from oestrogen-rich women being donated to oestrogen-poor women, in a splendid example of the ultimate in socialized medicine.

However, with growing acceptance of the logic of HRT and growing demand for it, sufficient supplies of human oestrogen were simply not available. Fortunately it was found that the structure of equine oestrogen so closely resembled that of human oestrogen, that women were able to metabolize it perfectly well, with no side-effects and with good relief of symptoms.

Just a few women, in my experience, are put off Premarin by the fact that it is derived from mares' urine. This is not really very logical since for so long insulin from the pancreas of pigs has been gratefully accepted for hormone replacement in diabetes. In medicine the success and safety of drugs is surely more important than the source.

However, in 1994 Premarin was attacked on rather different grounds by the Animal Rights movement, who insisted that the collection of the urine involved cruelty to the mares and foals.

Back in 1972 when I was making my own enquiries, I was assured that the special herds of mares, contracted to supply the urine required, all ran free on the Canadian Plains, doing what comes naturally to become healthily and happily pregnant. At that time, when Premarin was the only safe oestrogen available, this was readily accepted.

As a result of recent complaints, however, the RSPCA and its American counterpart undertook a close investigation and reported that although conditions generally were good, they felt the mares were confined for over-long periods for urine collection and that foals were separated too early from their mothers. The makers noted the criticisms, and agreed to take steps to remedy both problems. Meanwhile, for any HRT users who remain worried or sensitive about the harvesting of Premarin, there is now a wide range of other natural oestrogen products to choose from.

Harmogen and Progynova have already been mentioned, but widely used now in HRT are others termed the 'free oestrogens', oestrone, oestriol and oestradiol, separate members of the oestrogen family, 'freed' and isolated from the others. Hormonin and Questrin are oral products that manage to combine all three in their tablets.

Where progesterone, the other female sex hormone vital for the combined therapy is concerned the choice is not so wide. Unlike naturally occurring oestrogens, the natural progesterone cannot be successfully used orally, as it is broken down by the acid of the stomach and not properly absorbed into the system.

Fortunately, progesterone-like molecules (called progestogens) have been developed, which are not destroyed in this way and which are successfully absorbed to perform the normal functions of natural progesterone. Those most widely used in combined HRT oral packs or included with patches in calendar packs are norethisterone, levo/norgestrel, medroxyprogesterone and dydrogesterone. The last of these marketed as Duphaston, has been shown in particular to give good protection to the womb, while not affecting the beneficial fall in LDL cholesterol induced by oestrogen.[2]

Where oestrogen is prescribed separately – not as part of a combined pack – some doctors prescribe the progestogen in the form of Primulet N (norethisterone), while others prefer to give Duphaston (dydrogesterone). The progestogen-only pill taken for just twelve days each calendar month is another good and acceptable way of providing the very low dosage of progestogen required.

Of course, that twelve days each month on the progestogen-only contraceptive Pill does not confer contraception and nor, as already noted, does any other form of HRT.

The wider choice of hormones and availability of blood hormone levels enable HRT today to be prescribed safely and varied to meet individual needs. But all drugs have side-effects for some patients, and this might be the place to list them.

The most common is a mild form of nausea, thought to be related to the nausea that occurs during pregnancy. The naturally occurring oestrogens appear to give rise to this far less often than synthetic oestrogens and the tendency can be minimized by taking the pills after meals. Even where such nausea occurs, it is usually only during the first cycle, or if the oestrogen dosage is too high.

Breast tenderness and swelling also sometimes occur and women who suffer from cystic mastitis can be more prone to this. Some others may experience just a little soreness, and decreasing the dose or the addition of progesterone minimizes all these problems.

As already mentioned, irregular, unexpected bleeding used to be the greatest disadvantage of oestrogen therapy, but regular use of a progestogen has successfully overcome this and disciplined the withdrawal bleed.

Sometimes weight gain and swelling may occur from water retention due to oestrogen, but again, this is more common with the synthetic oestrogens. As mentioned earlier, the many studies now done have found weight gain to be linked to ageing rather than HRT.

There may be also slight darkening of the nipples and surrounding area, and occasionally some slight pigmentation freckles on the face. Changing the brand of oestrogen can eliminate this tendency too.

Finally oestrogen naturally promotes cervical secretions, and although this is desirable and far preferable to abnormal menopause dryness, it can sometimes be excessive, and again, this can be controlled by reducing the dosage, or adding a progestogen.

Most women will not incur any of these side-effects, but where they do the wider choice of medication now available certainly means that by selecting the correct preparation and varying the dosage and regimen, it is almost always possible to find a form of HRT to suit the individual patient.

Many studies have been done to compare the positive results achieved with various oestrogens, and even more interestingly to compare them in double-blind trials against a placebo.

A placebo (from the Latin verb, to please) is simply the name given to an inactive substance, such as chalk or water, which will pass through the body with no biological effect, but which is disguised to look like some actual medication.

The term 'double-blind' indicates that neither the patient nor the doctor is aware at the time whether the placebo or the real medication is being used, though coded records enable this to be established later when it is time to compare results.

Because someone taking a placebo *believes* it is a medicine, there is often a so-called 'placebo effect', and the patient does actually feel better – proof of the influence the mind and the thinking can have on health.

It has been fashionable in some quarters to insist that many menopause symptoms are 'only in the mind', and in such cases clearly a placebo should work just as well as an oestrogen.

In practice, however, the many double-blind studies carried out have disproved this. One done by Professor G. Lauritzen and quoted at the 1972 Geneva Workshop Conference on HRT, was fairly typical. Several hundred menopausal patients were involved, and although on the placebo the expected percentage felt better, the percentage whose complaints actually disappeared was nil. In contrast on estriol (1 mg) 68 per cent of symptoms disappeared, and on conjugated oestrogen (1.25 mg) 92 per cent disappeared.[3]

One would hope that this sort of result would have disposed for ever of the belief long cherished by some men (and regrettably by some doctors) that menopause symptoms are largely psychological, a miserable nervous reaction induced in middle-aged women by the prospect of loss of fertility and loss of youth.

Where a woman's life, her interests and her sense of identity and importance have centred exclusively around either her fertility or her physical beauty, it is true the loss of these may well aggravate the menopause and other problems of ageing.

But basically menopause problems are not psychological – they are physiological and can be pathological – they result from the deficiency of oestrogen and they respond to treatment with oestrogen. They do not respond to chalk coated with sugar.

Chapter 12

The implant technique

Until the advent of the 'patch', the implant technique was the only way in which oestrogen could be introduced directly into the bloodstream, giving a slow, steady release at low dosage and closely simulating ovarian function.

The method consists of inserting a pellet of natural oestradiol into the subcutaneous fat of the abdomen or buttock. The procedure takes only a few minutes but provides oestrogen protection for up to six months! A local anaesthetic makes the process painless, and the optional extra of a testosterone pellet can be popped in at the same time for any woman needing a boost to her libido.

It was on my second visit to the United States in a private clinic in Augusta, Georgia, that I saw the implant system used for the first time. My research and reading of the medical literature on the menopause and HRT made it clear that there was one doctor whom I had to see – Robert Greenblatt, Professor of Endocrinology at the Medical College of Georgia.

Not only was Dr Greenblatt one of the top endocrinologists in the world, and the man who for eighteen successive years had contributed the section on endocrinology to the year book of the *Encyclopaedia Britannica*, but he was also a top gynaecologist and pathologist. The combination of these disciplines had led him to do major work on infertility, where his development of the drug, Clomiphene, had brought him a crop of gold and silver medals, and most recently the French Order of Chevalier of the Legion of Honour.

But in addition to this, Robert Greenblatt had also for many years been a leading exponent and advocate of hormone replacement at the menopause, and my visit to Augusta was timed to coincide with a conference on the Management of Ageing, arranged at the University under his auspices as President of the prestigious American Geriatric Society.

With doctors flying in from all over America, with his own house guests and his own lectures scheduled, I was a little dubious about how much time he would manage to spare me. I need not have worried. On my first morning he joined me with other doctors for breakfast at my hotel before 8.30 a.m., so that we could talk before the official programme started. This sort of energy and dynamism was just as evident in his approach to HRT, and spilled over into the charisma from which his patients clearly drew immense confidence.

His position regarding HRT was very simple.

A basic premise in endocrinology is to restore hormonal balance (he explained). Oestrogen deficit after the menopause should be relieved just as much as thyroidal, pancreatic, or adrenal deficits, and it should be replaced by oestrogen, not by homespun psychology or tranquillizers. How can either of these be expected to arrest a deteriorating metabolic milieu? And why should barbiturates, bromides and tranquillizers, so foreign to the human organism, be preferable to natural oestrogen?

Dr Greenblatt estimated that 75 per cent of women become acutely oestrogen-deficient within a few years of the menopause, and believed HRT should be offered to every woman with symptoms and even to those without, if an oestrogen deficit is present. In particular he insisted that even in the absence of any other symptoms, the presence of osteoporosis is sufficient reason to initiate therapy with small doses of oestrogen (along with increased calcium and protein intake and exercise) for the rest of the patient's lifetime. He told me, 'Oestrogens appear to apply a brake to the parathyroids' capacity to stimulate bone resorption, and in severe osteoporosis, oestrogens protect by minimizing further skeletal deterioration and collapse of vertebrae'.

For oral HRT, Dr Greenblatt always used conjugated oestrogen, Premarin, the only natural oral oestrogen then available. He favoured continuous administration but insisted on producing a cyclic effect and regular shedding by interposing seven-day courses of progestogen alongside oestrogen. This is the basis now of most modern combined products, except that the progestogen course has been extended to twelve days for greater womb protection.

Like Sir John Peel, he was convinced about the importance of using progesterone. He insisted,

Where you are going to give oestrogen in full replacement dosage to a woman with an intact uterus, there should be a functioning, secreting endometrium. Oestrogens alone can produce complications such as painful breasts, weight gain, irregular bleeding and hyperplasia (abnormal thickening of normal tissue). All this is avoided and bleeding disciplined with the use of a progestagen, and with such a safeguard, I believe it is correct to keep the oestrogen continuous to avoid recurrence of symptoms and increased resorption of bone, that otherwise would occur during the week when oestrogen is withdrawn.

Where patients were unable to accept monthly bleeding, Dr Greenblatt prescribed a lower dose of Premarin (usually .625 mg) for five days, then a two-day break. Such short cycles, designed to avoid breakthrough or withdrawal bleeding, would not these days be considered to offer high enough overall dosage for adequate bone protection.

For their convenience, because so many patients came to him from great distances, flying from as far away as San Francisco, Zimbabwe and Canada, Dr Greenblatt made considerable use of the long-lasting implant technique. He explained to me, 'Sometimes these patients come from areas where there is no local doctor able to supervise Hormone Replacement. The implant method confers six months' trouble-free replacement, and the slow-release mechanism is particularly effective'.[1]

On my second day in Augusta, I was given the chance to judge this for myself. Suitably clad in a white coat, and with the permission of each patient, I took my place with the medical team working with Dr Greenblatt at one of his private clinic sessions.

On that day there was the usual broad spectrum of problems a gynaecologist and endocrinologist must deal with. In particular there were many young women with infertility problems, and I was lucky enough to witness the happiness of one girl and her husband, when they learned that after a course of Clomiphene the on-the-spot pregnancy test and examination confirmed conception. It was a great moment for us all.

As well as infertility, there were cases of frigidity also responding well to hormone treatment, and there were several young patients being treated for problems of growth.

However, it was the varied crop of menopausal cases, both surgical and natural, which were of special interest to me. As it happened on that particular day, they were all on return visits, and so the usual six-monthly check-up was done, with internal examination and smear tests. The slides were examined by Dr Greenblatt there and then under the microscope to confirm the level of replacement was correct and that the vaginal mucosa was healthy. Once this was established, a repeat implant was done.

This proved a very minor surgical procedure and quite painless. First a shot of local anaesthetic was injected into the lower abdomen, and then immediately a small metal tube was inserted in the same area, down which the appropriate hormone pellets were introduced. The tube was withdrawn, a piece of sticking-plaster applied and that was that. It took only a few seconds, though the effect would last for up to six months.

In some cases along with the oestrogen pellet or pellets (each 25 mg of pure estradiol), Dr Greenblatt also inserted a pellet or pellets of male testosterone (75 mg) and he explained,

I have found the administration of testosterone along with the oestrogen enhances the benefit, frequently in eliminating depression while improving energy and sex drive. There is also often considerable improvement in any arthritic condition, but the unexpected bonus has been in relief of migraine-type headaches. While oral HRT relieves these in approximately forty per cent of cases, the ratio rises to about eighty per cent with the implant system.

I asked Dr Greenblatt about the risk of virilizing effects, such as facial-hair growth and deepening voice which has been associated with the use of male sex hormones by women. He was reassuring about this and told me,

The excessive use of testosterone in the past has given rise to fears about this and to some condemnation of doctors who prescribe it. As much as 25 mg of testosterone propionate was sometimes prescribed per week for up to six months, which meant a woman was taking in all 600 mg over the period. But with the implant method, a pellet only contains 75 mg, and this is released slowly over the same length of time, adding up to only one-eighth of that dose. Even where two pellets are required, it is still only one-quarter of the dose.

From his thirty-five years' experience, Robert Greenblatt estimates only between 5 per cent and 10 per cent of women may show some slight virilizing effects, and then it is usually only a small increase in facial hair. If this does happen, such patients have the option of discontinuing the testosterone, when the hair growth usually recedes. But Dr Greenblatt told me that most of the few women affected prefer to still continue the treatment because they feel so well on the combined therapy. He explained, 'They are often women who, after surgical or natural menopause, have suffered almost total loss of libido, which this treatment has restored. The male sex hormone does not change the direction of sex drive, but it does intensify the response'.

Dr Greenblatt made the point that for many women oestrogen replacement alone is enough to restore sexual feeling.

It eliminates dryness, makes the vaginal mucosa softer and more succulent and ensures proper lubrication, and this all means that sexual relations become easier and more enjoyable. This in itself brings a marked improvement in response. But where oestrogen alone fails to achieve this, then testosterone should be added. It can also be given orally in the form of methyltestosterone at 2.5 mg per day over short periods. Again if virilizing reactions start to occur, it is simple to discontinue treatment.

Only one out of the six patients I saw and talked to, who were having testosterone implants, had developed a facial hair problem. She was an attractive brunette of about thirty-five who had had her ovaries removed and who admitted she had always been a slightly 'hairy' type. Although Dr Greenblatt did suggest she might like to forgo just one of her testosterone pellets, she refused, 'My husband is happy the way things are,' she explained. 'We have a great sex life and I can get the hair growth dealt with quite easily'.

Because I had already met so many women on oral HRT, I chose particularly to talk to those receiving implants. Another one was Gail McCuan, aged twenty-seven from South Carolina, who had had both ovaries removed some years before.

Pellets of oestrogen and testosterone were implanted even before my operation so I never suffered any drastic symptoms afterwards. But I soon notice when the action of the implants begins to decline toward the end of each six-month period. Then I get tired and depressed and have no sexual response. But within a day or two of the new implants, I am back to normal and feeling fine.

Another patient who talked to me very frankly was Mrs Leonora Holtzman, who had flown in from Miami, Florida. Fifty years old, blonde and attractive, she looked far too young to have two grown-up children and four grandchildren. She told me,

After a hysterectomy at the age of forty-one, I had a terrible time. I had fearful sweats every night and awful depression. The worst part for me was my inability to cope with life. At that time my children were giving me a lot of problems, and when I finally flew to Georgia to see Dr Greenblatt that first time, I remember telling my husband that if this doctor could not help me, I would not come home . . . and I meant it. I was really at the end of my tether. My doctor back home had told me that I needed a psychiatrist and I had begun to believe him. But the hormone replacement revolutionized my life. I've been coming back ever since for my two testosterone and one oestrogen pellets. With me they only last four months, probably because I lead such an energetic life. I feel so well and full of energy now, that I am even tackling the job of bringing up my seven-year-old grandson.

Mrs Evelyne Thorpe from Athens, Georgia, was another patient who had been on implants for ten years, in her case to counteract a severe natural menopause. Aged fifty-six and a widow, she received no testosterone, just two oestrogen pellets. She told me,

Before treatment I suffered terribly from hot flushes and

night sweats that left me drenching wet. After the first
implant the symptoms disappeared completely. Now, even
if I didn't have my next appointment fixed, I'd know when
the six months was up, because I begin to feel exhausted
and that is the signal that the implant is running out. Within
seven days of having the new implant I feel energetic and
well again.

Implants are, of course, also available in this country.
They were initially pioneered here by London gynaecologist, Mr Scheleyer-Saunders, but were never widely
used in Britain until after John Studd, today one of our
leading experts in HRT, went to America to look at Dr
Greenblatt's work and then came back to carry out his
own extensive research and trials at the NHS menopause clinics he then ran at Dulwich and King's College
Hospitals in London.[2]

His authoritative, well-published studies have confirmed the effectiveness and convenience of the implant
method, particularly for busy women. One of them,
Teresa Gorman, MP for Billericay, recently made
public her own use of HRT and the fact that she now
favoured the implant method.

I feel it is so iniquitous that women often have to fight their
way through the hostility of GPs for this treatment that I
decided to come out with my own experience. I'd seen how
much my American friends benefited from HRT and I
went to the Menopause Clinic at King's and got the
treatment there. That was nine years ago. I started with
the oral treatment and then went on to implants. The results
have been outstanding. The aches and pains I'd been
suffering in my wrists went and my old energy came back.
Now I can keep going from seven in the morning often to
one or two a.m. if the job demands.

I also know HRT is preventing the wretched bone loss
that occurs after the menopause. Once gone it's never
recoverable and I believe helping to prevent osteoporosis
alone makes HRT worthwhile.

The implant method also improves libido and if that

means that a previously happy marriage stays happy then that's another jolly good reason in its favour.

Their cost, bearing in mind that they last for six months, is only slightly more than for other methods and they are increasingly used under the NHS, especially at the time of surgery for removal of ovaries.

In the past, British gynaecologists did not always favour the idea of immediate oestrogen replacement at the time of surgery, because of perceived thrombosis risk. But with this fear now totally dismissed so far as *natural* oestrogen is concerned, the use of natural oestradiol implants at this time should be mandatory. Unless any of the very few contra-indications to HRT exist, there is no excuse whatever for any woman being left after surgical menopause without the benefit of this form of prompt replacement technique.

A hospital that led the way in this was the John Radcliffe, Oxford, and a report on this aspect of their work was given at the 20th British Congress of Obstetrics and Gynaecology, which I attended in London. Details were presented of a comparison carried out of two groups of patients after bilaterial oophorectomy. Each patient in one group had received an implant of 100 mg oestradiol 17B (Organon) at the time of the operation. Women in the smaller group had received no implants. There was a striking difference in their subsequent experience.

Eleven of the fourteen patients in the small group with no implants developed severe flushes, and five of them required oestrogen therapy. None of the twenty-three patients with an implant seen in the first fifteen months after surgery had hot flushes at all. Only one of another fifteen patients with implants seen between sixteen and twenty-four months after surgery had developed mild flushes, as had two out of four patients examined after twenty-four months. All three of these women dated the onset of flushes to approximately eighteen months after the operation, indicating these particular implants as effective for between one-and-a-half and two years.[3]

Advocates of the implant system point out that the concentration of hormones required is only about one-third of the dose needed by the oral route, and also that implants avoid any untoward gastric or intestinal side-effects, which can sometimes occur with hormone tablets taken by mouth. They claim also that psychologically the patient is not continuously reminded of her condition by having to adopt a daily pill routine.

This avoidance of the need for daily tablet taking can certainly be an advantage where the patient is either not sufficiently motivated to remember, or sometimes is simply incapable of remembering.

Some doctors maintain that there is no advantage in using implants, except where other HRT methods are not well tolerated or where testosterone is also required. Certainly the patch, which also releases the hormone directly into the bloodstream, is a simpler way of achieving this physiological form of delivery. Just a few women, however, do find they get skin irritation with any type of patch.

Apart from the fact that the dosage cannot be so easily adjusted or swiftly changed as with the Pill or the patch, the main disadvantage for most women is that implants cannot usually be done by a GP, and so involve visiting a specialist NHS clinic or going to the private sector.

Another complication which can arise for some women on implants is something called tachyphylaxis. This is not some terrible disease, but the name given to a build-up of tolerance to the original dosage. This results in implants being needed at decreasing time intervals to maintain relief of symptoms. However, if these are given earlier for this purpose, it has been found that in a few cases it leads to the levels of circulating oestradiol rising above the normal range. To avoid this, most gynaecologists now prefer to do a routine check on hormone levels *before* inserting a repeat implant earlier than scheduled. A neat solution to bridge the time gap and relieve returning symptoms is temporary resort to a low-dose patch.

With this problem so easily solved, implants are likely to remain popular and often seem the choice of very busy women and those in public life who may have a lot of travelling to do, with difficult hours or other pressures which interfere with a set routine.

This applies very much to women in show business, who are obvious candidates for HRT anyway, as they depend so much on appearance and vitality, not just for personal success but for professional survival.

Films, television and stage work make tremendous demands both physically and mentally, and no middle-aged actress can afford to put a production or her own career in hazard by allowing herself to fall victim to hot flushes, lack of memory or lack of energy, all of which are so often part of the menopause.

Although from the time it first became known and available, a great many stars have taken advantage of HRT, there used to be considerable reluctance to admit to using it, rather as there still is today to confess to cosmetic surgery. It seems as though admitting that you are combating any form of ageing is tantamount to admitting that you *are* ageing.

One pleasantly forthright star, who had no such inhibitions and who was only too happy to tell me she had used Premarin for some years, was Canadian-born Barbara Kelly. She looked young enough to persuade anyone that HRT works, and meeting her again on a TV programme in 1991 after a gap of nearly twenty years, I found little change in her appearance and none in her zest and energy.

Another actress ready in the early days to admit to being on HRT was Jean Kent, then a star of stage and screen on both sides of the Atlantic. She talked to me frankly about her own attitude to female problems:

A woman's biology is very important in my business.

Menstruation affects the voice. An opera singer never sings at that time – her programme is always arranged to avoid that. But the menopause can be even more of a problem. Once the ovaries start to pack up and you are no longer fertile, there is no doubt nature loses interest in keeping you attractive. Also hot flushes can be terrible things. When it started with me I went straight to my gynaecologist, and once he was convinced it really was the change of life, he put me on hormone implants.

I don't believe in suffering unnecessarily either from a personal point of view or, of course, from a professional one if I feel my work is going to suffer too. Acting does require good health. Television imposes long rehearsal hours, with clothes-fitting often having to be done in the lunch hour because of tight schedules. Films involve starting in the make-up room at 7 a.m., and you will have to look as fresh at 6 p.m. as you did in the morning. The stage is more a matter of a few hectic hours, but these are in front of a crowded house and use up more strength to the minute than films or television put together. HRT has maintained my stamina.

The cost of an implant done privately is in the region of £75; but it must be remembered that this lasts for six months. The cost to the NHS is considerably less than this, of course, though still more than for oral HRT or the patch.

Despite this slight hitch, implants are likely to remain popular; not only are they highly effective, but convenient, too, especially suited to anyone who has had a hysterectomy because without need for a progestogen there is no bother with pill-taking. Implants often seem the first choice for very busy women.

I find it an interesting sign of our more open times that, in contrast to 1975, when it was extremely difficult to get, VIP women are more than happy to talk about HRT and to record all the many benefits it has brought them. Marjory Proops, Sue Lawley, Dinah Sheridan, Kate O'Mara and Jill Gascoine are just a few who have hit the HRT headlines.

Those who claim to know insist Mrs Thatcher was also on HRT for many years, and certainly both her appearance and stamina during a long, demanding term in office would support that.

The royal users, of course, are properly discreet about such matters, but both the Queen and the Queen Mother publicly supported the Great British Bone Appeal, launched in November 1989 by the National Osteoporosis Society, to help finance their work for HRT and for better management of the established disease. The two royal cheques were among the first to be received.

Support from the top carries considerable influence and breeds growing confidence in HRT, as other women see that those who can afford the best advice use this treatment. But even more reassuring is the fact that over half of all female doctors opt for replacement therapy when they hit their own menopause. These are women in the very best position to judge the pros and cons.

It was a 1996 survey by the National Osteoporosis Society (NOP) among women doctors which established that 51 per cent of them used HRT and 41 per cent stayed on long term. These figures were compared to the take-up rate of only 18 per cent among other women, with only 6 per cent continuing long enough to reap the benefit conferred on heart, arteries and bones.

So what is it that keeps our prescribing rates too low? What is stopping more women from benefiting from HRT?

Chapter 13

Present problems and future hopes

There was a time when the low level of HRT prescribing in this country could be laid fairly and squarely at the surgery door, with too many family doctors refusing to prescribe. Instead they clung to outdated medical school teaching, which decreed that the menopause did *not* require treatment, and that the degenerative effects that followed were an inevitable part of ageing in a woman.

The flood of despairing letters I received in the 1970s and early 1980s amply confirmed this problem. Women wrote complaining that their GPs not only refused to prescribe HRT themselves but refused the referral letter needed to attend menopause clinics or consult a gynaecologist.

One woman, who inadvisedly waved my book around in the surgery, described how her GP had flung it furiously into his waste-paper basket. Another wrote, 'My doctor not only refused to consider oestrogen replacement but, when I asked for a referral letter, actually said "I forbid you to go elsewhere." '

When Queen Victoria was faced with reluctant doctors, objecting to her insistence on the new chloroform being used to ease a royal birth, she is reputed to have royally clinched the argument with the words, '*We* are having the baby; *we* shall have the chloroform.'

It is tempting to feel that, even without such royal authority, women wanting Hormone Replacement and faced with uncooperative doctors, should try exerting similar female firmness and insist, 'We are having the menopause; we shall have the Hormone Replacement.'

Unfortunately assertiveness on the part of the patient has never been very welcome to doctors. They have been too concerned with preserving the old mystique surrounding medicine – so necessary when it had little else to rely on; and the old autocratic attitudes – so fitting in the days when they were perceived as the wise men in a largely uneducated community.

Today it is a very different situation. Increasingly effective modern drugs and sophisticated techniques make the preservation of medical mystique not just unnecessary but unrewarding. What modern medicine demands for maximum efficiency now is an *informed* patient in partnership with an approachable and communicative doctor. This is being recognized today in the new emphasis being placed on the training of doctors in communication skills, and in the new encouragement the rest of us are receiving from the Department of Health towards greater responsibility for our own health and a partnership role with our doctors.

All this is leading in the right direction, but tends to overlook the fact that many doctors, under the pressure of busy NHS surgeries, simply cannot give time for the full discussions this requires.

Where HRT is concerned, successive surveys have certainly uncovered a regrettable communication gap between some doctors and some patients. In recent surveys women repeatedly complained of not being given sufficient information by their GPs – this applied particularly in the North of England and in Scotland, both areas with low HRT prescribing rates.

One large NOP study, based on face-to-face interviews in their own homes with over a thousand women, aged forty-five to fifty-eight, randomly selected for geographic area and socio-economic status, found that among those who were aware of HRT at all, only 30 per cent knew that long-term treatment prevented osteoporosis, and a mere 3 per cent that it protected against cardio-vascular disease. This would help to explain why this and other surveys found that two-thirds of users stayed on HRT for only somewhere between six months and a year.

A lot of the women in this group had curtailed treatment simply because the obvious symptoms worrying them had been relieved, so they saw no point in continuing. Another 20 per cent had come off because of side-effects, with breast tenderness most often quoted. Even more had stopped treatment because of the inconvenience of enforced periods.

Despite massive media coverage in recent years, the same NOP survey revealed suprising basic ignorance. Over half of the women questioned did not know that the cause of the menopause was failing ovaries and falling oestrogen levels. Small wonder then that the whole logic of replacement therapy eluded some of them, with a quarter of those who refused HRT perceiving it as 'against nature'.

Where HRT is rejected on these grounds, it would help if doctors would just explain that what is really against nature is for women to live so long today – long enough for the degenerative effects of hormone deficiency to seriously affect the quality of life.

The biggest disincentive to taking HRT, however, confirmed in all recent surveys, is fear of a possible link with increased risk of breast cancer. Although one in two women dies from a heart attack or a stroke and only one in twelve dies from breast cancer, it is the latter that most frightens women, and repeated inaccurate scare stories in the media do nothing to help.

GPs, of course, if they have kept up with the latest research findings, should be able to reassure their patients by putting the small (and still unproven) increased risk of breast cancer into perspective, setting it in the context of HRT's proven ability to reduce coronary artery disease, the biggest killer of all, by 50 per cent, and to virtually eliminate osteoporosis.

Fears about HRT safety simply do not fit the pattern

of worldwide statistics that show *mortality* rates from all cancers (including breast cancer) to be actually lower in women on HRT, and women on replacement therapy to live two years longer on average than untreated women.

Although prescribing rates for HRT have risen from the 8 per cent of the mid-1980s to between 15 and 20 per cent in the mid-1990s, doctors argue that they should be going up faster and further, insisting that at least a third of women who are eligible would benefit from replacement therapy.

Far from being reluctant to prescribe, or refusing HRT when asked, most GPs today offer it without *waiting* to be asked. What they are *not* always offering, however, and what these surveys show is most wanted, is reassurance and fuller information. Women need a clear explanation of the basic concept and of the importance of long-term protection, together with details of risk, benefit, side-effects, and the wide variety of HRT products and methods available.

In the 1990s 'The Communication Challenge' became a subject I was asked to cover both in talks I was invited to give to doctors and in articles I was asked to write for the British Menopause Society and the International Health Foundation. This seemed an encouraging sign that at least the problem was being recognized and addressed.

But if closing the communication gap is a challenge for doctors, there are others for women. On an individual level a very few may still have to face obstinate doctors who, against the trend, refuse to prescribe them HRT.

In such cases today a well-argued approach can usually cause opposition to crumble. A casual mention of knowing that HRT has been officially advocated by the Royal College of Physicians *and* the Department of Health is a good starter. If necessary this can be followed by a tactful reference to the protection you understand HRT gives against osteoporosis, heart attacks and strokes.

It is hard to see how any doctor faced with such a well-informed patient can risk refusing treatment. If he or she does, then there are two alternatives – either change your doctor or exert your right to a second opinion. It is an accepted credo that a patient who is not happy about diagnosis or treatment has the right to ask for this.

The relevant clause in the Health Service rules states that the services a doctor must give shall include 'arranging for referring patients, as necessary, to any other services provided under the Health Service Acts'. These services embrace all forms of specialist consultation, but obviously, the crux lies in the interpretation given to the words 'as necessary' and *who* decides what is necessary.

As professionals doctors may feel they are better equipped to make the decision. But in relation to the menopause in particular, it can be argued that only the woman herself can really judge how important it is for her to get relief of immediate miserable symptoms or how necessary to look for long-term protection.

The *Patient's Charter* and the latest partnership concept both make it unlikely today that a doctor will refuse a referral letter, but under the rules of the National Health Service it is not in order for a patient to try to consult a specialist direct.

Fortunately, where HRT is concerned there are a few accepted avenues of self-referral. One is through the admirable Amarant Trust which runs its own private clinics and help-lines. Some other private clinics will on occasion take patients without the usual letter from their doctor, on the understanding that the GP will subsequently be informed of any treatment prescribed.

In the old days many family planning clinics, then run by the FPA itself, offered both menopause advice and HRT to their patients. Since they were handed over to local authorities in the late 1980s, this has no longer been the case, but FPA headquarters, Women's Health Concern and the National Osteoporosis Society can all supply long lists of clinics which help women to find one in their area.

The addresses of these organizations are given at the back of this book together with a similar list of clinics, coded in this case to show those which are purely private, those private but subsidized and those which are NHS. It must be stressed that it is never possible to guarantee such lists are complete or that all the clinics on them still function or retain the same status – old ones close and new ones open all the time. One way or another, however, *all* women in this country today should be able to get HRT, and hopefully few will have to battle for it as they did in the very recent past.

The broader challenge for women, and one which needs and deserves their support *en masse*, is that of getting area health authorities (AHAs) to comply with vital Department of Health recommendations to provide better services for early osteoporosis detection and treatment.

In 1995, a DOH special report on osteoporosis laid this responsibility on all area health authorities, but an NOS survey eighteen months later found that over half of them had done nothing; 42 per cent provided a very minimum service, while 62 per cent still had no overall strategy for tackling a problem that will inevitably worsen as our ageing population continues to increase.

The most scandalous finding in the survey was that only 12 per cent of AHAs were meeting the most important DOH recommendation – to fund bone scans for women at high risk of osteoporosis. Until they do so, expensive capital equipment continues to lie idle. Over half of all health authorities actually possess bone densitometers, but only a quarter of them provide the necessary funding for these brilliant machines to be set to work, so that thinning bones can be detected early and appropriate treatment started in time to prevent painful, disabling, and sometimes lethal fractures.

The cost of setting up such a basic clinical service in one health area is estimated to be only around £50,000 – *less* than the Authority incurs in dealing with local hip fracture incidents over just a two-week period.

The costs of HRT and of bone scans for women at high risk of osteoporosis, whether borne by the health authorities or shared with budget-holding GP practices, are always going to be less than the cost of dealing with the serious end results of prolonged oestrogen deficiency – osteoporotic fractures and coronary artery disease.

Another challenge women and their doctors might tackle successfully together is the basic injustice of the government imposing a double prescription charge on combined HRT. The great majority of HRT users have not had a hysterectomy, and safety demands that for them both hormones must be prescribed. Yet this mandatory combined treatment attracts two separate charges. Many doctors recognize the unfairness of this and include several months' supply on one prescription form to reduce the overall cost.

If a GP does not or will not do this, women can reduce costs to some extent themselves through the prescription season ticket system. This poorly advertised service brings some saving over the four-month or twelve-month period allowed, but for a lot of women it may not be easy to fund such one-off payments.

The fact that the more recently introduced Continuous Combined version of HRT, containing the same two hormones but taken together daily, attracts only a *single* charge points up an absurd anomaly. This muddled situation cries out for pressure to be put on government to set one single prescription charge for all HRT packs.

Britain, of course, is struggling to operate a National Health Service, inadequately funded and staffed, within a limited economy already drained by extensive social and welfare commitments. In these circumstances, there is currently little option but to adopt a system of stern priorities. Serious illness, urgent operations and life-and-death matters are dealt with in the main promptly and efficiently; expensive equipment, X-ray procedures, tests, biopsies, anaesthesia, surgery and drugs are all supplied free of charge.

This has meant all too often that while preventive medicine wins fine words, in practice is gets only low priority. Some forms, of course, do earn a well-deserved place within the NHS structure. Free contraception is one, justified not only in terms of greater personal and family stability, but as an aid to better economic planning. Vaccinations against polio, typhoid, diphtheria, measles and whooping cough are also provided as routine and free preventive medicine, often organized via school clinics.

I believe there is a strong argument now for better preventive medicine and screening later in life, and the argument becomes stronger as the ratio of older people in every population continues to grow. Prevention is not only better than cure: it is cheaper.

More than a quarter of all women in the developed world are post-menopausal. Ten million of them live in Britain, each with a life expectancy after the menopause of another thirty years. The magnitude of the public health challenge this presents should not be underestimated. One answer might lie in special clinics for the older woman, offering menopause counselling with HRT and referral for bone scans where appropriate, targeting in particular those who have had a hysterectomy or ovaries removed in the past, *without* benefit of oestrogen replacement.

Such a clinic could also liaise with other specialist centres. It seems to me that mammography services, for instance, should when possible be routinely extended to the over-sixty-fives, instead of this important check-up being provided only for the older age group if special application is made. The risk of this disease does not diminish with age and, until any possible HRT/breast cancer link is finally ruled out, GPs should certainly be doing annual palpations for every woman on HRT, with referrral for a mammogram every two years for those who have been on this treatment for more than a decade.

Not least of the services clinics for older women might offer would be some pick-up on patients, who have never had a cervical smear or who have not had one done for many years. Professor Josephine Barnes, past President of the Royal College of Obstetrics and Gynaecology, and Britain's leading woman gynaecologist, made a good point regarding such screening in her own advocacy of HRT. She pointed out to me:

Hormone Replacement Therapy brings immense benefits, but it will bring even more if it succeeds also in persuading women to have regular vaginal and cervical smears. Those who are at present reluctant to come forward for a check-up specifically to preclude malignancies, might respond much more readily in the wider context. Women must be educated to avail themselves of these forms of preventive medicine.

Dr Greta Malmberg, the seventy-three-year-old doctor already mentioned as a long-term user of HRT, and who worked in school clinics, added her own views on this. She said, 'We already have family planning clinics, pre-natal clinics, ante-natal clinics and school clinics. It seems to me it is time we also had special clinics for the mature woman'.

Such services are already in existence attached to NHS hospitals, usually fragmented into menopause clinics within gynaecological departments and breast screening done in X-ray. The snag, as we have seen, is that to get access our British system requires an all-important referral letter from a doctor. In this respect Britain differs not only from most European countries including France, Germany, Spain and Italy, but also from America.

Comparing the American and British systems, I found any advantages in the States, both in regard to HRT and more general medicine, seemed largely confined to those lucky enough to possess a good deal of money or incomes sufficient to permit adequate private health insurance cover. In either of these cases, the system of private medical practice permits the great boon of freedom of choice, not just in selecting a doctor, but in selecting *the* doctor for the job at the time of most need.

With no compulsory referral or registration, and with their professional plates clearly indicating specialist interest and knowledge, there is no problem for the American woman in finding a doctor or gynaecologist to prescribe replacement therapy, providing she can pay for it or is covered for it by her medical insurance.

Most of the women I met got their HRT in this way, but it was a different matter for the very poor. Those on social welfare qualified for free medical care, but how often this would include something like HRT varied from state to state, hospital to hospital, and even doctor to doctor. Whereas urgent medical treatment was provided and the bill taken care of by the state in the case of the really under-privileged, a therapy more concerned with the quality of life than preservation of life seemed less likely to be provided.

Between the very poor on social welfare (those qualifying for free medical services) and the middle-income group, who wisely went in for medical insurance, there was a strata of people on low incomes, who did not qualify for free medical treatment and who gambled on continuing good health, because they could not or would not budget for insurance payments. Their predicament highlighted the disadvantage of voluntary rather than compulsory health insurance, because without spare money and without insurance cover, I found medical help was sometimes sought too little and too late.

It remains to be seen if efforts to bring in a form of compulsory health insurance in America can succeed in closing the gaps in medical care and still retain valuable freedom of choice. The rejection of Hillary Clinton's elaborate and seemingly over-expensive plans suggest it is not going to be easy.

Meanwhile, as mentioned earlier, the American system, like any other system of private medicine, does involve a degree of pressure on the doctor to comply with the patient's wishes. Otherwise both patient and fee simply go elsewhere. If a doctor has real grounds for believing the treatment a patient wants is actually wrong or harmful, it becomes a choice between maintaining his/her professional integrity or his/her bank balance.

On the question of the risk of exploitation of the patient by the doctor, which British medicine appears to see as the great danger of a purely private medical system, the opportunity for this most certainly exists. I can only say that, in my own admittedly limited experience of American medicine, I did not find evidence of it being very widespread.

Obviously, in all countries and systems, there will always be some doctors prepared to abuse the high ideals of medicine by allowing the art of healing to become subordinate to personal gain. But merely living the other side of the Atlantic, or practising in a country where socialized medicine is limited, does not suddenly turn good doctors into bad ones or men with ideals into unscrupulous predators.

To an English woman, used to subsidized drugs and free medical care (or more properly medical care which *seems* free because payment is concealed within National Insurance deductions), the costs of keeping healthy in the USA could certainly seem pretty high. But I found many instances of compassionate doctors adopting an almost Robin Hood attitude, with payments from rich patients being quietly used to subsidize care for the poorer ones.

The problems of availability of HRT, of how it can be obtained and financed, will no doubt be solved in different ways in each country. But behind the different medical systems and solutions all over the developed world, the same pressures are at work.

There is the pressure of numbers, of the increasing *quantity* of women living on long beyond the menopause. And there is also the pressure of *quality*, of the fact that increasing numbers of educated women, doing interesting and demanding work with feet firmly on the career ladder, want and expect to be kept fit enough and energetic enough to go on doing this work. There is the pressure of communication, of the fact that these increasing numbers of educated women can read, hear and see features on HRT, know it exists and believe it can help them.

For their own sakes, for the sakes of their families and for the sake of society itself, much more needs to be done in the field of positive health to extend the period of mental and physical vigour for men and women. And this has to begin by ensuring a healthy middle age, for that is the time when most of the chronic diseases of later life begin.

Even on existing knowledge and research results alone, HRT has proved to be good preventative medicine, not just against the immediate menopause symptoms, but in the long term against some of the important chronic disease – against those of the cardiovascular system, of the nervous system, probably against some forms of malignancy, osteoporosis, some types of arthritis, and against prolapse and incontinence, the scourges of women in old age.

With so many advantages proven, HRT research needs now to concentrate on resolving the few questions that remain. Further work is needed to confirm if HRT really can reduce the death rate from bowel cancer, something suggested in a study involving many thousands of women and reported in 1996 in the *Journal of the National Cancer Institute*.

More work is required to see if the beneficial effect of oestrogen on Alzheimer's disease can be consistently reproduced. And research must continue to establish *if* HRT in the long term does increase the risk of breast cancer and to what degree. Only then can a final balance sheet be drawn up on the value of HRT.

Medical tradition is against rapid change, hostile to innovation, and, no doubt, on balance we should be grateful for this. Only reasonable caution and pains-taking research and testing can ensure that tragedies like the thalidomide one are kept to a minimum.

But caution can be carried too far and this often seems to be the case where new ideas to improve the purely female lot are concerned. It must seem almost unbelievable to doctors today that in the middle of the last century women were allowed to go on suffering and dying from puerperal fever for twenty years after Zemelweiss had effectively demonstrated that this infection could be eliminated by the now obvious pre-caution of properly cleansing the hands before an internal examination. Doctors could not accept such a simple but new concept, even when by using this basic hygiene Dr Zemelweiss reduced the deaths in his own obstetric ward from 11.4 per cent right down to less than half of one per cent.

Maybe it will seem equally unbelievable in another twenty years that women in the 1990s were still suf-fering and dying from the effects of post-menopausal osteoporosis, when simple replacement therapy could have saved them. HRT, though it came late to Britain, has been in increasingly wide use now for nearly fifty years, and the contraceptive Pill with its own essentially more powerful oestrogen content, for almost as long.

Significantly, during all that time, despite the increased usage of oestrogen this represents, there has been no parallel increase in breast cancer, and cancer of the uterus has declined. In contrast, the incidence of lung cancer has soared in women, reflecting their increased use of cigarettes.

One American doctor, Francis P. Rhoades, of Detroit, Michigan, suggested in the *Journal of the American Geriatric Society* back in 1967 that male doctors could have a special reason for being slow to accept a treatment that made the female menopause obsolete. He urged:

The physician should not let inherent male resentment of female longevity and biological superiority deter him from his medical responsibility. Those who regard the menopause as God's will should critically re-examine the traditional goals of their profession. Because men do not experience the dramatic and often devastating changes represented by the menopause, they have come to regard it as normal for women to suffer the consequences of cessation of ovarian secretion.

All splendid ammunition for Women's Lib! But I cannot believe that in many cases this sort of resentment has really been at work. I can believe that apathy has, and to some extent this has been the fault of women themselves. Far from making too much fuss about the menopause, in the past we have made too little.

If every woman now genuinely suffering from a miserable menopause took herself to her doctor, made him aware of her problems and emphasized the risk of osteoporosis she could be running if she did *not* receive HRT, I believe any lingering apathy towards the menopause would collapse.

At a recent medical conference one doctor argued publicly that in the face of the current osteoporosis statistics and with HRT known to prevent this condition, it amounted to 'criminal negligence' for any of his medical colleagues to withhold this treatment, in particular following a surgical menopause.

The growth in HRT usage, and the readiness of more

and more GPs to prescribe, stems not only from their increasing confidence in its safety, but from the wider choice of products and methods that now allows them to tailor treatment more closely to individual need.

But if doctors are to do this, selecting the most appropriate form of HRT for each patient at each stage of the climacteric, medical schools will have to give fuller initial training in this area of medicine, with regular refresher courses arranged to keep GPs abreast of new techniques as they develop.

With ever more sophisticated concepts in view, the future of HRT looks bright. Improved oestrogens and progestogens are currently being developed directed at specific targets and effects. Improved delivery systems are coming along all the time with the combined patch already in wide use. A new way of introducing progestogen is just coming in, using a coil (or IUD). This is inserted into the uterus where it gives slow release locally of small doses of hormone, so that the amount of each bleed is kept to a minimum and there is also a reduced risk of PMS-type symptoms, which plague some women during this phase of the cycle.

Medicine already has tablets which release their content very slowly, but at the moment this slow release is limited by the time the tablet can spend in the gut. But it may prove possible to coat the hormone at a molecular level, so that it is released into the bloodstream over prolonged periods, perhaps to allow a once-a-month tablet.

In the longer term, there may be a prospect of ovarian transplants or even artificial ovaries. Already the chemical reactions performed in the ovaries to produce their oestrogens are known, and eventually artificial substances may be used to synthesize these hormones *within* the body when the natural ovaries cease to function.

Alternatively, the genetic engineers may some day be able to locate and cancel the vital switch which instructs the ovaries to shut down.

But most of this lies in the future. In the meantime, I believe the young women of today, used to their daily hormone contraceptive Pill, will find that by the time they reach the menopause, it will be equally accepted for them to be given the lower dosage of hormones that will eliminate the problem failing ovaries can bring. It will be as natural to combat these aspects of ageing as it is now to get eyes tested, and to be given a prescription for the right lenses. Replacing hormone deficiency at the menopause will be as automatic, as it now is to replace thyroid deficiency or give insulin.

And maybe when the words 'Women's Lib' are no more than the remembered echo of some old battle-cry from an ancient victory, the words 'Biological Lib' will continue to have meaning for women as the basic freedom, designed not to decry the female role, but to control and maintain it.

Appendix 1

Mail witness

Letters from my postbag recounting the experiences of ordinary women and ordinary families caught up in the miseries of the female menopause provide more convincing evidence than any words of mine, both of the dimension of need and the degree of help required. They also reassure other women that they are not alone in facing certain problems at this time, and this in itself can provide a form of comfort.

The bulk of my mail comes, of course, from British women and most of the early letters bear graphic witness to the difficulties once experienced in the UK in obtaining HRT. But over twenty-five years they have changed, reflecting the progress that has been made. Menopause problems are still described but usually as past problems, with women now just taking the trouble to let me know how HRT has helped them and how well they now feel. To better trace this progress, the letters selected for inclusion in this edition have been set in rough chronological order, with the later letters being most relevant to the situation today . . .

So this Appendix is not written by me. It is written by many different women, most of whom I have never met, but all of whom I thank. A great many of them would have been quite happy for full names and addresses to be published, but others were shy about this because often they had written freely about intimate problems. So it was decided to standardize presentation and in general merely use an initial and a place, and also obviously to publish only the really relevant extracts.

'How can we get our doctors to take us seriously? I am an ordinary NHS patient, aged forty-three years with three children. I am far from being a hypochondriac and have rarely visited my doctor, except for the babies, in years. Twelve months ago I went to him to tell him I have never felt so dreadful in my life and felt sure I was suffering from some obscure disease. He just laughed and said I was a healthy colour for a corpse.

'Two months ago I went back again, mentioning that I felt physically weak, very depressed and at least twenty years older (my husband says I look it). This time I was told "it was just my age and nothing could be done". I wasn't given any advice so came home and read an ancient book on the menopause. My husband is younger than me and very fit and all this is not helping our marriage. He puts great reliance on medical advice, and if the doctor says there is nothing wrong with me, my husband believes him. Please, where can I get HRT?'

Mrs W., Bordesley Green

'... Why is it we can read about these things which sound just what we need, but if we ask our doctors they would probably say they have no time for such trivial things? They give the impression they have really sick people to attend, and anyone worrying them about the menopause is just neurotic.

'My periods stopped at thirty-nine and for eight years I have felt upside down and sometimes have felt like suicide. I feel I have nothing to live for and I really touch bottom. My skin has aged and hairs grow round my mouth and chin. Believe me, this is not just vanity, although I suppose I do want to look better, but most of all it is the terrible depression that really knocks me flat and the awful headaches.

'I am not a neurotic. I am just a woman who has

brought up three children, two are university students.
I live in a council house, have a job and a decent
husband, but I would just like to know how people like
me can get the sort of help you write about.'

Mrs M. N., Essex

'While living in Canada four different doctors there
prescribed natural oestrogen and it was excellent for
me. Since returning to the UK and running out of
tablets, I have been absolutely up against a stone wall.

'My GP does not agree with it at all and regardless
of my well-being and the fact that I have been so well
on it for so long, utterly refuses to prescribe. It is the
more maddening because I know from enquiries at
the local chemist that the oestrogen I was on, called
Premarin, is obtainable, but only on prescription.

'I have been made to feel positively humiliated for
wanting to stay well and attractive at my age. Yet in
the small town where we lived in Canada, prior to
moving to Montreal, all my friends of my age were
benefiting from replacement therapy and that was
seven or eight years ago now.'

Mrs F. D., Devon

'I am forty-eight and have started the menopause and
get so depressed. I've been to my doctor over hot
flushes and sweating and sleeplessness at night, but he
doesn't take much notice, just says it is natural and
gives me tranquillizers to keep me quiet.

'I have a job in an office and three children, the
youngest only nine years old, and a dear good husband,
whom I love very much but our sex life is rapidly
becoming nil because I feel so awful. Please can you
help me?'

Mrs M. V., Worcestershire

'Some years ago we rented our house to some Ameri-
cans and the women were horrified to know that no
provision was made to give replacement hormones to

middle-aged women. I am a State Registered Nurse and have four children whose ages range from two to fourteen. Over the last two years my menstrual cycle has been disturbed; I suffer from pre-menstrual tension and have put on weight around my hips. When I asked my previous GP for some hormones, he told me he believed in the natural menopause, so I did not go again.

'I would like to consult a gynaecologist on a private basis because I have a husband who is very active sexually, and I do not wish to spoil our lives or those of my children with a wife and mother who is under strain. I consider it is much cheaper to treat this condition at this stage rather than let it develop further.'

Mrs S., Berks

'Since the onset of the menopause life has been very grim. I am being woken at night with palpitations and night sweats and also suffer from a type of migraine. I have seen my doctor but get no relief from the treatment he has given me, although I take as many as twelve pain-killing tablets a day.

'The depression and apathy I feel are affecting both my marriage and my job, which carries a great deal of responsibility.'

Mrs M. P., Essex

'I am fifty-seven and ceased menstruating seven years ago. I suffer with frequent hot flushes which make me feel terrible, but I also have a very peculiar sensation, a really horrible feeling as though something is moving through my veins – I find it hard to explain, and if I ever mention it to my doctor, he only laughs. He has never even asked me about going through the "change".

'My query really is: Have you come across anyone else with this sort of symptom? It makes it worse not being able to convince my doctor or explain how awful it feels. You mentioned on the programme that there

are some special clinics. Could you tell me how to find
out about them?'

Mrs H., Birmingham

'A gynaecologist has put me on hormone replacement.
I have been feeling much better, but every time I go
to my local GP for the tablets, he warns me that not
enough is known about long-term results and whether
it can produce cancer, which I am sure is no doubt very
laudable, but naturally it disturbs me. Could you put
me in touch with someone who has been on this therapy
for a long time, to reassure me? My GP has made me
very nervous but I feel so well, I just can't give up and
go back to the misery of hot flushes and sweats.'

Mrs K., Herts

'... Like a lot of women I have a doctor who seems to
feel that Librium and anti-depressants are the answer
to all female ailments at this particular time.

'From having a happy married life and being an
ordinary individual, over the last three and a half years
I have become an anxious, irritable, moody, introspec-
tive *thing*. Because of continual irritation in the vagina,
intercourse has become a memory, and when my
husband and I went together to see our family doctor
we were told, "There's nothing I can do about it" I
have a really wonderful husband, but the feelings of
utter frustration loom larger than life at times. At fifty-
three sex is not the vital thing it was when we were
twenty-one, but it was always there, but now the discomfort amounting to real pain and the lack of help
from the doctor whom I thought could help, has meant
our sense of humour like our relationship has become
very strained.

'I find it very hard to believe that the present "me"
is the same woman who used to sing over the housework, enjoy the family and friends and not have to
wonder how things will be in the morning. Will it be
an up or a down day? I wouldn't have believed the

"change" could be just that – transformation is a better word.'

Mrs L., Ilford

'After a hysterectomy at the age of forty-eight, when I looked only thirty-eight, I was afflicted with hot flushes every ten minutes day and night. My husband retired to his own room and my marriage was finished. From then on I aged rapidly. My skin dried up and my hair thinned. I get desperately tired. After the operation I know that I must lack hormones, but my doctor will not give them to me.'

Mrs L., Canterbury

'Thank heavens I found your book! The last eighteen months had been hell with night sweats so that I couldn't sleep, palpitations, painful muscles and a crawling under the skin. At times I felt faint, dizzy and almost disembodied with ears ringing and awful headaches. The storms of weeping were quite dramatic and my depression really bad. I looked terrible. Intercourse was painful and I was just lucky to have a fantastic husband who put up with me.

'I started the change five days after my fortieth birthday, nearly two years ago. My mother had started hers at thirty-nine and now has very brittle bones. She fell recently and broke her arm and shoulder and cracked her ribs. Her menopause was as terrible as mine but in those days nothing could be done.

'After reading *No Change* I began a long battle to get HRT. There are six doctors in the practice, five men and one woman. I was told to pull myself together, that I was too young for the change and that HRT was not any use as it was all natural and I must put up with it.

'I finally told the woman doctor that if I couldn't have a trial course of HRT I was going to go privately. It was only then that she agreed to it and even told me she had lots of ladies on the therapy and recommended it! How hypocritical of her. Still, I achieved my objective so I don't really care.

'I am now on my second month of HRT. The difference is unbelievable. I look good again. I sleep all night. All I've got left of my misery is the odd headache and some breast soreness. I am hoping that after the three month trial period is up it will all have faded to a nasty memory. Your book really has helped so much. Thank you for writing it.'

Mrs. C. S. R., South Humberside

'I am forty-nine and have been a widow for seven years. My indecision and foreboding for the future increased over the seven years rather than receding. I made many bad decisions. To this, in the last twelve months, were added severe joint pains, dizziness, crying bouts, sleeplessness, tiredness and formication.

'After three months of Prempak I am restored to the energetic, decisive, sensible, painfree woman I used to be. I didn't have to persuade my doctor – *she* suggested HRT to me. Because I was still menstruating (albeit irregularly) I had assumed I didn't need it. I suppose living alone and without a family to notice how affected you are, these menopause symptoms just creep up.

'I am a councillor representing an area of high unemployment and with one of the highest death rates in this country. If the over-worked, over-stressed women I represent don't get HRT at source – i.e., the GP – they are too tired, too poor and too "menopausal" to seek it elsewhere. For years contraception was the monopoly of the middle class – I intend to do what I can to make sure this doesn't happen to HRT.

'To admit to any experience of hormonal disturbance is still considered a sign of weakness by many men and some women. For that reason I must remain anonymous.'

A Metropolitan Area District Councillor

1st letter

'. . . While I am grateful to the Press for bringing such treatment to my notice, please, what is the use if we are unable to obtain it?

'It is now nine years since I first read about HRT in an American magazine and since then I've had five years of the menopause with all the miserable physical symptoms and depression. I have written to every magazine and paper carrying articles on HRT asking where I can get help, but only get the usual reply – medical etiquette forbids them giving doctors' names.

'Finally I was lucky enough to find a Canadian doctor working in this country who examined me and put me on oestrogen. The change was miraculous. However, after one year, he left and returned to Canada, and his successor refused to continue the therapy. He gave me a prescription for sedatives which I have not even had made up, and patted me on the head as if I were a senile old dear. So here I am again – insomnia, backache, deep depression, the lot! Can you please help? Don't refer me back to my own doctor, as I assure you he will not even discuss it.'

2nd letter

'Thank you so much for details of the clinics. I got an appointment and was given the most thorough examination I have ever had; blood tests, urine, heart, lung, the lot. Above all, it was wonderful to be spoken to as if I were an intelligent human being, instead of a neurotic menopause freak.

'I am now on natural oestrogen and feeling better already. I simply cannot understand the attitude of so many doctors. My original GP never even used the word menopause, but simply told me to get my family to help me over the depression. He made me feel to admit to the menopause was like admitting to being "queer", that it was something which should not even be discussed.'

Mrs A. B., Lancashire

'I work full time in a large and busy school as well as looking after my home, my husband and a twenty-year-old son. I am only forty-four but the menopause seemed suddenly to hit me with "hot waves' so frequent and severe that I would wake up at night soaking. This, coupled with mild cystitis (which I had never had before) was making my life at school and at home very difficult. Now only after a couple of months on 1.25 mg Premarin, it is wonderful to be entirely free of flushes and feel normal and healthy again.'

Mrs W., Birmingham

'... I am a State Registered Nurse and my work is demanding. From Prempak I am finding great benefit. I am on a twenty-eight-day cycle with one week off. There are no side-effects and it seems to have given me a great deal of energy, although I only heard of it and started on it later than recommended and well after the menopause.

'Judging from my experience and observations over some years of working in geriatrics, I am strongly of the opinion that if the treatment could be made available on the National Health at the right time, much of the degeneration and suffering of old age could be retarded and alleviated.'

Mrs G., Oxfordshire (State Registered Nurse)

1st letter

'I am writing to you in sheer desperation. I can see no future for myself and recently tried suicide, so that my family, my son and my husband, could be free of their trouble and worry about me. My son has just left home, to share a flat with a friend, and I know this is the thing to do nowadays, but I wonder if it has to do with my behaviour.

'I am fifty and with the onset of the menopause, have felt like an old woman, having to give up my job because I could not cope with it as well as my home. Sex is not only painful, but I have no interest in it

whatever. My husband and I read your article in *Good
Housekeeping* and he said, "This is just you – this is
what you need."

'My doctor says there must be some reason for my
breakdown (his term), but there is nothing more than
I have set out here. My doctor has been giving me up
to fifteen pills a day, but apart from making me sleep
better, there is no improvement. Recently I have been
so miserable I have taken my consolation when alone
all day in whisky. I have told my doctor of this, and been
sent to a psychiatrist who specializes in alcoholism.'

2nd letter

'Within a few days of receiving your letter I got an
appointment at the clinic. The gynaecologist examined
me and said he would be able to help me. I am now
taking the HRT tablets and already feel much better.
I am to go again in a month's time and then again in
three months.'

Mrs K., Nottingham

'... A year ago I wrote to you in great distress
explaining that when I was forty-five I had my womb
and ovaries removed, and since then had been in a
most miserable state. I was not given hormones but
only barbiturates which did nothing but made me feel
giddy. All my doctor would say was that I had to expect
it at my age. But you don't like to feel you've had it at
fifty. Anyway after your letter I went to the gynaecologist and he put me on HRT. I felt I must let you know
how much better I feel. I can manage my housework
again and that awful heavy feeling has gone. I am so
grateful and must apologize for not writing before. My
husband made me write to you the first time because
I was in such a state that my marriage and the whole
family were suffering. He wants me to tell you what a
difference the treatment has made to all our lives.'

Mrs S., London, E.7

'I am a nursing sister and cheered you on in your radio talk, nodding full agreement with all you said. From personal experience I know replacement therapy works. I have been on 1.25 mg Premarin for six months and feel terrific. Now I advise all my apprehensive post-gynae patients that if they can't get oestrogen replacement they must change their doctor. I had to bombard my own GP before I got it.'

Mrs G., Tonbridge

'There is no doubt reading *No Change* and managing to get help from the Birmingham Menopause Clinic has made my life worth living again. I had the most miserable few years as my doctor was quite unconvinced about HRT, but seeing the tremendous good it has done in my case, he is now prepared to prescribe for other patients and to supervise my own treatment. It's reassuring to find doctors can at least keep an open mind and supply the necessary referral letter and be big enough to admit later that they are not omniscient. He has become a complete convert.'

Mrs J., Birmingham

'After reading *No Change* I plucked up courage to ask my own GP for hormone replacement, and to my amazement there was no problem. He insisted that I should go on the combined therapy and warned me that this would involve a regular withdrawal bleed, but I can honestly say I feel so well on the treatment that I count this a very small price to pay. I intend to stay on just as long as he will allow me to do so and I gather this may be some years as he believes it protects against osteoporosis.'

Mrs S., Sheffield

'Since my doctor put me on Cycloprogynova I have had no further flushes and my sleeping has improved. I really feel energetic and intercourse which had become painful is now once more part of our married life. My

husband says I am a "new woman" and that is the
way it feels after months of feeling a prematurely old
woman.'

Mrs B., Cardiff

'When my husband presented me with an updated 1988
version of *No Change* in a Coventry bookshop on Sat-
urday, I decided I must write to you again and tell you
once more how grateful I've been for your wonderful
response to the letter my husband, Vincent, wrote to
you twelve years ago when, after removal of both
ovaries, I suffered such severe depression that I spent
six months in a psychiatric hospital. It was all useless
and it was when they said they could do no more that
Vincent took the initiative of writing to you.

'Since going on Hormone Replacement Therapy, as
you suggested, I feel I have gone from strength to
strength. As I mentioned in an earlier letter, we went
on to adopt three children and have led a normal,
happy married life ever since.

'I continue to take two tablets daily, each 0.635 milli-
grams. After we moved to Leicestershire last March my
"new" GP did suggest that I should halve the dosage. I
did this but after six weeks I had definite joint and
muscle pains, with pins and needles in my arms, severe
headaches (hitherto practically unknown) and a feeling
of lethargy.

'As my blood pressure has always remained normal,
I have reverted to the old dose of two tablets daily and
the muscle pain is now negligible and I feel fine.

'I am now sixty-one and can truly say I feel happier
and healthier than I did when I began teaching at
twenty. At fifty-nine I was asked to accept responsibility
for an unruly class of thirty-three children and I was
able to rise to the challenge for two years until we
moved to this area. Since then I have done continuous
supply teaching and, this week, have been offered a
teaching post for the next two terms.

'Your original copy of *No Change* had to be replaced

because it is still "on loan" to a person who is loth to return it. I don't blame her and I'm happy for her to have it.'

Mrs J. B., a vicar's wife, Hinckley, Leicestershire

'I thought you would be interested to know that two generations of my family are now benefitting from HRT. I was only twenty when I heard you on radio and bought a copy of *No Change* for my mother, who was suffering severe menopause symptoms following a hysterectomy. After reading it, she asked her doctor for HRT but he refused to prescribe. In the end she persuaded him to refer her to the Birmingham Menopause Clinic, where she was put on Premarin and within weeks her symptoms had all gone.

'Recently, at the start of my own menopause, I bought the new edition of *No Change*, which indicated things were now much better and it was great to find when I went to my GP and mentioned my own menopause symptoms, he at once suggested HRT. He also told me about the patch and within weeks of using them I've not only got rid of my flushes but got back the energy and confidence I seemed to have lost. My doctors emphasized the long term benefits as you do in your book and I intend to stay on HRT as long as I can.'

Mrs S., Solihull

'When my periods became irregular and I began to have flushes, I went to my doctor and he recommended HRT. I felt better within only a week or two and have gone on feeling really well for three years. But then I read an article about the increased risk of breast cancer and soon after saw a TV programme which also mentioned this. As a result I came off treatment and now my flushes and night sweats have come back together with bad depression, something I've never had before.

'My doctor was reassuring and suggested that if I was still worried I should get your book. I did find it very helpful and have gone back on treatment. My physical symptoms disappeared again very quickly but it took over two months before the depression went. Life again seems worth living and I plan to stay on treatment this time. I have told myself that having mammagrams in due course will serve as a check on breast cancer.'

Mrs B., Bristol

'My GP group run a Menopause Clinic as part of their Well Woman service and I found it a great help recently talking to other women who had experienced menopause symptoms and had them relieved by HRT. I had always thought that getting through the menopause was just a matter of being strong minded, but it hadn't worked for me. I found flushes and night sweats made me so tired and irritable that the whole family were suffering. Talking to the other ladies there, and then to my doctor, decided me to try HRT and it has been like a miracle. I am back to normal and only regret now putting myself and my husband through that year of misery.'

Mrs V. M., Swansea

'I am fifty-seven and had suffered from backache for several years before last December, when I finally sustained a vertebral fracture. In the next five months I had four other similar fractures one after another. As soon as I recovered from one, I went down with another. I was virtually an invalid and for a time felt totally helpless and dependent. After osteoporosis was firmly diagnosed, I spent four weeks at the Royal National Hospital for Rheumatic Diseases, where I was put on HRT and given exercises regularly – three times a day.

'I have had to be on sick leave from my secretarial job and can only hope to return part-time. I still find it difficult to bend and do simple things such as get out of bed or wash and dress, and have to be very careful not to knock myself as my bones are very brittle and will still break easily.

'Because of my spine crumbling so badly I have lost five inches off my height. Osteoporosis has affected every aspect of my life and it could have been so different if I had known about HRT in time to prevent it.'

Mrs J. L., Batheaston

Appendix 2

Statements and quotes from doctors

'In previous editions of this book I have expressed sadness that so many women with miserable menopause symptoms were being denied HRT at a time in their lives when they needed all the help they could get. In 1996 I'm happy to report that the majority of doctors are now convinced of the benefits of HRT and most recognize that while HRT can relieve most of the distressing symptoms associated with the menopause, perhaps its real value lies in the long term protection it offers.

'However, the "HRT message" does not always seem to get through to women and I still find many who are not aware of the long term benefits and even more surprisingly some who are not even aware of HRT at all. To this end, the UK needs to embark on a major public relations exercise to bring the benefits of HRT to the attention of all women. In this my GP colleagues have an important role to play, particularly in situations where patients, who would very much benefit from treatment, continue to be alarmed unnecessarily by media reports of adverse complications. In particular women still worry about a perceived increase in the incidence of breast cancer, without realizing that any such increased risk, if it exists is small and confined to those women who continue on oestrogen for fifteen years or more – in any event such slightly increased risk of breast disease is far outweighed by the benefits which HRT confers to the cardio-vascular system and in protecting against osteoporosis. Indeed, one of the major breakthroughs in the last two years has been the realization that the administration of HRT to women who have been treated for breast cancer does not appear to affect adversely the long term prognosis. So, thankfully we are now in a situation where we can offer HRT with safety to these patients.

'All too often I hear woman say they are reluctant to use HRT because "it is not natural". Personally, however, I would argue that the post-menopausal women who uses oestrogen is keeping her body as near natural as possible, and it is the woman who is not using oestrogen who is in the unnatural state.'

J. A. Jordan MD, FRCOG, Consultant Gynaecologist and Medical Director, Birmingham Women's Hospital

'Research in the medical field is traditionally more concerned with pathology than with normality. This certainly holds good for the climacteric and the post-menopausal age. In no phase of life, however, is the line between what is normal – and therefore acceptable for the individual – and what is pathological – and therefore unacceptable – thinner than here.

'Finding a solution for the problems of these ages is a medical responsibility, because it is medical science which has prolonged life and, in doing so, has called the climacteric and old age into existence.'

Dr L. Jaszmann, Department of Obstetrics and Gynaecology, Regional Protestant Hospital, Bennekom

'When I started the first HRT clinic for the menopause in Birmingham twenty-five years ago, I ran into a lot of medical and media opposition which resulted in the clinic being closed down for three months following protests from the local branch of the British Medical Association.

'Although never far from controversy it is now accepted that HRT is a major advance in preventative medicine, but the challenge is that so few women, only around 15 per cent, actually take advantage of this therapy. Yet the evidence is overwhelming that HRT prevents many heart attacks, strokes, and fractures, while also helping depression, bladder function and sex life. What is more it has been shown that women who have enjoyed long term HRT live almost two years longer than those who have not.

'Despite these important benefits, unfounded anxiety about HRT causing weight gain is allowed to dissuade many women from treatment with this, oddly. This is the most common reason given for not going on HRT. Others include fear of breast cancer, the inconvenience of periods in some cases accompanied by premenstrual type symptoms in the progestogen phase.

As non-bleed treatments become established, women will increasingly have the benefits of HRT without such problems. But full acceptability will probably only occur as women are offered a wider choice of oestrogens, dosage and various routes of administration. These are becoming available – a year ago there were only ten HRT preparations, in 1996 there are thirty-five.

'As regards fears of increased breast cancer risk, we have a responsibility to get at the truth of this story, but at the moment it seems to me more likely that there may be a greater pick-up in HRT users but not necessarily a greater occurrence. All studies except one have already shown a much decreased mortality from breast cancer in HRT users compared with non-users.'

John Studd, Consultant Gynaecologist, Chelsea and Westminster Hospitals

'I think that our duty is to help our patients to live under optimum conditions. We have, with oestrogens, reached the stage where we know what benefits such a therapy may have. We know a lot about the risks, perhaps not everything. We should not forget that abstaining from oestrogen therapy might harm the patient, and that is also a risk.

'On the basis of our present knowledge of the beneficial effects of oestrogens, it would be wrong to deny these effects to the big group of women in the post-menopause.'

> *Professor V. Madsen, Gynaecological-Obstetrical Department, Gentofte Hospital, Copenhagen, Denmark*

'Innumerable clinical observations indicate that oestrogens are not only beneficial for the physical symptoms and affect the reactions in autonomic nervous system, but also improve the entire emotional state in the climacteric.

'They relieve general symptoms, such as weakness and fatigue, and purely emotional components, such as anxiety, tension, mood depression and irritability. Furthermore, a great many patients report a general feeling of well-being as a result of oestrogen treatment. The symptoms are rapidly or gradually relieved depending on the individual response and the hormonal drug dosage used.'

> *Dr H. Kopera, Department of Pharmacology, University of Graz, Austria*

'In the normal way the proper place for prescribing HRT is within general practice, and selectively used it proves exceptionally rewarding for both doctor and patient. Prescribing the lowest dosage of oestrogen to relieve symptoms combined with a regular 10–12 day course of progestogen each cycle (or using one of the already prepared packs) the supervision required is only comparable to that of oral contraception.

'The patient successfully established on HRT gains a noticeably improved quality of life, and far from increasing the GP load HRT tends to reduce consultations otherwise sought for a variety of physical and psychological problems associated with the post-menopause.'

> *Dr T. C. G. Smith, Ayrshire*

'It is important to decide whether one should aim at

prophylaxis or treatment. By the time one treats osteoporosis, for example, a considerable amount of bone has already been lost. It is a case of shutting the stable door after the horse has gone. It is not quite the same as treating the atrophic vagina. Once this has developed one can get a good and quick result with oestrogens. The practice of medicine, as a whole, tends nowadays to be more and more a prophylactic type of medicine. I do not think we should just treat a condition when it arises; we should think more about prevention. That is why I would argue strongly in favour of replacement therapy in connection with the bone disease.'

Dr J C. Gallagher, MRC Mineral Metabolism Unit, General Infirmary, Leeds, United Kingdom

'Every woman, sooner or later, undergoes inevitable ovarian senescence.

'This phase, the climacteric, is not something she endures for a few months, or a few years, but for the remaining days of her existence – during which time she may well be considered a physiologic castrate.

'The difficulties of the menopause – the imbalance of the automatic nervous system, the psychogenic disorders and the metabolic disturbances – continue, from mild to severe form, until the end of life. It is unrealistic to withhold measures that may make the transition smoother or prevent disabling pathologic processes.

'Since sex steroids became available, their value in relieving menopausal symptoms is generally acknowledged. There is, however, no unanimity among physicians as to who should be treated or why. At one extreme, the therapeutic nihilist believes the menopause is a physiological phenomenon which must be managed by reassurance and the use of sedatives or tranquillizers. At the other extreme, others feel that every post-menopausal woman should be given oestrogens, regardless of the presence or absence of symptoms. We think that a more prudent attitude is somewhere between, and that oestrogens are most beneficial in the management of correctly screened patients. No other drug or therapy is able to relieve a menopausal woman of her many discomforts so completely.'

Dr Robert Greenblatt, Professor of Endocrinology,
Medical School of Georgia, USA

'Oestrogen is a fundamental hormone in the total physiology of womankind. We have focused our attention too much on the effect of this hormone on the reproductive apparatus without giving adequate attention to its total effect on all body tissues.

'The physician has a responsibility to the growing numbers of post-menopausal women in our society. With proper treatment these women can stay youthful, useful, healthy and happy. Properly administered oestrogen replacement therapy will provide a feeling of well-being and eliminate many post-menopausal problems.'

Dr J. Parks, Professor in Chief, OBGYN, George
Washington University, Washington, DC, USA

'It is only a question of when and to what extent each woman will become a victim of this insidious (oestrogen) deficiency blended with chronologic ageing.

'Many women may be restored from a chronic state of semi-invalidism to mental and physical health with the judicious use of ovarian steroid therapy. It is unrealistic to withhold measures, before or after the menopause, that can make life pleasant and prevent crippling and disabling pathological processes.'

Dr W. G. Francis, Chief, Dept. of OBGYN,
York-Finch General Hospital, Toronto, Ontario,
Canada

'Long-term replacement therapy with oestrogen for complete gonadal failure is far more rewarding (than short-term use for symptomatic relief) and should be continued indefinitely to retard the physical atrophic changes and the development of degenerative metabolic disorders. This is an exciting area of preventive medicine which will help women to retain their good health in their advancing years.'

Dr M. E. Davis, Joseph Bolivar DeLee Professor Emeritus of OBGYN, Univ. of Chicago, Illinois, USA

'Oestrogens generally will relieve all symptoms (of atrophic vaginitis) within a short period and transform the red mucous membrane into a pale, healthy vagina.

'Oestrogen also plays an important role in maintaining the pelvic supports of the uterus and bladder, as well as the mucus membrane of the bladder. The summation of these effects is to preserve all of these structures in a healthy condition, as they are during the reproductive years, and to reduce the frequency of cystitis, stress incontinence, and prolapse.'

Dr E. J. DeCosta, Professor, OBGYN, Northwestern University School of Medicine, Illinois, USA

'For our middle-aged women, accustomed to cyclic administration of natural oestrogens and the added utilization of ana appropriate progestogen, there will be no climacteric with its menopause. For these women, in fact, for almost every woman in the civilized world, the climacteric and menopause are unnecessary, totally obsolete. Our older ladies will avoid osteoporosis and their bones will not break. Non-shrivelled breasts and genital organs will be taken for granted. These women will be infinitely more pleasant to live with . . .'

Dr Robert Wilson, Consultant Gynaecologist, New York

'Many physicians believe that endocrine therapy during menopause affects primarily the autonomic nervous system reactions, not the psychiatric symptoms. I disagree. Oestrogens improve the entire emotional state of the patient.'

Dr Dorothea Kerr MD, Payne Whitney Psychiatric Clinic, New York

'We cannot promise our ladies that oestrogens will restore them to everlasting youth – but we can assure them they will be healthier, happier, more vigorous, and more contented members of our society.'

John Walsh, MD, Washington, DC, Clinical Professor of Obstetrics and Gynaecology, Georgetown University Medical School

'The climacteric syndrome is unique to the human. In no other species in the animal kingdom do we find the complex of symptoms and findings that are seen in the menopausal female. It may well be that the human female, because of the advances of medicine, now lives much beyond her reproductive potential.

Consequently she is then exposed to the exigencies of ovarian oestrogen deficiency. It is for this reason that we feel that the climacteric syndrome, whether presenting with or without symptoms, warrants continuous long-term oestrogen therapy; thus one would treat the oestrogenic-deficient female in much the same way one would treat a thyroid deficiency whether or not there is a presenting symptomatology.'

Herbert S. Kupperman, MD, Ph.D., Gynaecologist, New York

'Prevention of osteoporosis is certainly high among the many known benefits of Hormone Replacement Therapy. Nothing in life is completely risk-free, but the risks of HRT (both known and hypothetical) are livable with and more than outweighed by the benefits for most women.

'As a result, it is my opinion that HRT should not be restricted to those women who happen to get hot flushes or similar symptoms just around the time of the menopause. There should be serious consideration of this treatment for *all* women and one really needs a reason for *not* giving it. The reason could be that she is unlikely to develop osteoporosis by virtue of her body mass or racial characteristics, or that she simply chooses to let nature take its course. But for many other women the *option* of obtaining the known long-term benefits of this treatment should not be withheld from them, as it sometimes is at present.'

John Guillebaud, Medical Director,
Margaret Pyke Centre

'I have used natural oestrogen and cyclic combined hormone therapy for patients over quite long periods, for as much as ten years in some cases. There is no doubt of its immense clinical benefit to some women between the ages of forty-five and fifty-five and does slow down some ageing processes for a time.

'No one should use oestrogen alone and without interruption day in and day out. Prolonged and continuous over-stimulation of the endometrium can be a factor in producing endometrial cancer. The important rule in oestrogen replacement therapy is that it must be intermittent and I believe the combination with a progestogen is a safer system.'

Sir John Peel, Consultant Gynaecologist, London

'In 1973 as a young Registrar I had the job of running the NHS Menopause Clinic opened at the Middlesex Hospital. That experience and seeing how HRT could improve the whole quality of life for women going through a difficult menopause convinced me then of the value of this treatment.

'Since those early days research in our British Clinics has established that using both hormones in the combined system of HRT is not only effective but also very safe. Well published figures feeding through from monitoring programmes show less uterine cancer in women on this treatment. They also confirm that HRT protects against cardio-vascular disease and we have long known that it protects against osteoporosis.

'In view of these proven positive benefits so clearly outweighing any possible risks, it is difficult to understand why any GPs now should be reluctant to prescribe HRT or continue to regard it as controversial. Yet as a consultant, I do still see women, both under NHS and privately, who have been forced to seek referral because a few GPs cling to outdated attitudes.

'Very often when GPs see these patients later, thriving on the treatment and taking on a new lease of life, this does more to convince them of the value of HRT than the many medical papers on the subject seem able to do. In most cases they begin to prescribe HRT themselves and find it very rewarding and easy to supervise.'

Peter Bowen-Simpkins, Consultant Gynaecologist,
Singleton Hospital, Swansea

'I believe there is a tremendous future in oestrogen replacement therapy. My concept is simple, and the passage of time will prove whether or not it is correct. Simply stated, I consider the climacteric, the menopausal period and the post-menopausal period to be manifestations of a deficiency disease. I use the term disease specifically to indicate that I do not consider it normal that women should be allowed to continue a life with the absence of a substance which is essential for their normal physiology. My analogy, one would not consider preventing patients with diabetes, mellitis or Addison's disease receiving the respective hormone replacement therapy, and why should we consider the menopause as anything less than a hormone deficiency disease.

'This particular philosophy is also based upon my belief that during the evolution of man, the onset of the menopause in the female of the species was not subjected to the forces of natural selection which have eliminated so many intrinsic metabolic defects.

'Obviously by the time the menopause had arisen the women had fulfilled her part in propagating the species. Indeed, it was quite rare for woman to reach an age where a natural menopause could occur. I think nowadays that one should differentiate between a pharmacological effect and a physiological effect, when one considers oestrogen replacement therapy, and with the wealth of evidence which suggests that no harm arises from the replacement of oestrogen in physiological dosages, I can see nothing other than benefit arising from the more widespread use of oestrogen replacement therapy.'

Dr Mansel Aylward, Clinical Research Consultant

'HRT is the only way to stop post-menopausal bone loss and, if it's introduced soon after the onset of the menopause, the bones will not get thin enough to fracture. This prevention of osteoporosis is all-important, as once bone is lost it's difficult, if not impossible, to restore. Normally the best one can hope is to prevent further loss.

'The earlier the menopause and the longer a woman spends in the post-menopausal state, the greater are her chances of developing brittle bones and fractures. For example, I have seen osteoporosis in a girl of twenty-nine just because she underwent her natural menopause prematurely at age seventeen. Thus, women who experience their menopause before forty, or perhaps even forty-five years of age, should be regarded as at particularly high risk. Because the post-menopausal ovary still makes a small contribution to the overall oestrogen status, where a woman has to have them removed and there is no contribution at all, preventive treatment in the form of HRT is mandatory. It should also be remembered that hysterectomy alone may sometimes compromise ovarian function.

'But however desirable it may be, it's still not possible to *impose* preventive treatment on all post-menopausal women. Some women and even some doctors may subscribe to the view that the menopause is "natural" but the development of osteoporosis is certainly not. Women should be made aware of the risks of the menopause and all should have access to HRT.'

John C. Stevenson, Consultant Endocrinologist, Wynn Institute for Metabolic Research, London

'In the whole of nature only the human female experiences a menopause, while other animals remain potentially fertile until death. Women today, with a long life expectancy of over seventy-eight years, can expect to spend on average one-third of their lives after the cessation of reproductive potential, in a state of ovarian failure and oestrogen deficiency.

'Fortunately the effects of hormone deficiency are now easily corrected by Hormone Replacement Therapy, and the eradication of night sweats, lethargy, dry vagina etc. can be very dramatic, and a rewarding experience for the woman, her family and the prescribing doctor.

'However, although these symptoms often significantly lower the quality of life, they are not life-threatening and no one ever died from a hot flush. But the long-term effects of oestrogen deficiency are a different matter. Osteoporosis can result in fatal fractures – those of the hip are associated with fifteen to twenty per cent mortality. Prolonged oestrogen deficiency can also increase the risk of cardio-vascular disease, while in contrast being on HRT long term has been shown to halve the risk of heart attacks and strokes.

'It is imperative that the value of HRT for the long term health of women should be more widely appreciated. Unfortunately, all too often the communication of medical matters to the lay public is either ill-informed, sensationalized or misleading. Hopefully, this book, by a journalist so well respected by the medical profession that she is frequently invited to talk at medical meetings, will stimulate much wider usage of HRT to help preserve the long-term quality of life for women.'

David Strudee, Consultant Gynaecologist and Director
of the Menopause Clinic, Solihull Hospital

'GPs are very aware of the suffering caused by osteo-porosis in older women. Prevention at last appears to be possible and the experience we have gained over the years in prescribing HRT to relieve the more obvious menopause symptoms means we are now ideally placed to implement its prophylactic use to help protect against osteoporosis and cardio-vascular disease.

'It was always recognized that this was particularly important following early natural or surgical meno-pause, but as it became clear that even where ovaries were conserved their efficient function could often be affected, we instituted a recall system via our Well Woman Clinic for women who have had this operation but whom records showed were not on HRT.

'Well-Woman Clinics in the practice setting are rapidly becoming universal, combining routine breast and cervical smear screening with measurements and recording of other parameters of health. This, together with increasing use of computers, means that all women can be offered regular screening. These clinics provide an excellent opportunity for HRT counselling as the menopause approaches, for identifying risk factors for osteoporosis and discussing treatment, as well as for regular monitoring of patients once HRT has been started.

'Our patients' greatest reservations concern the long-term safety of HRT, particularly with regard to breast cancer. GPs look forward to the reassurance of large long-term studies to discount these fears and to combat the often ill-informed interpretations of medical reports in the lay Press.'

Mark Vernon-Roberts, General Practitioner, Swansea

'My personal view of HRT has swung over the years from cautious scepticism to acceptance and now to enthusiasm. Unlike the event on the road to Damascus my personal conversion has taken place over a period and is based on the scientific evidence which has emerged in that time.

'In our practice clinic, we now actively contact women and encourage them to embark on HRT and a range of preventive measures which have been shown experimentally to reduce the incidence of osteoporosis. An account of this clinic has been published in the British Journal of General Practitioners.'

Jean Coope, General Practitioner, Macclesfield

'Over the last ten or fifteen years, major advances have been made in our understanding of both the short and long-term sequelae of oestrogen deprivation at the menopause. There is overwhelming evidence that HRT is not only the best treatment for distressing meno-pausal symptoms, but also our only means of preventing osteoporosis and it's tragic consequences. Perhaps even more important than this, however, we know that oestrogen replacement has a significant role to play in the prevention of arterial disease in women, reducing substantially the number of deaths from heart attacks and strokes. Arterial disease is the major cause of death amongst women in this country, outnumbering deaths from cancer of the breast, uterus and ovary combined. Thus HRT has the potential to make an enormous positive impact on women's health, both for individuals and for society as a whole.

'There is a growing awareness among the general public that the problems of the menopause are con-siderable, but can be overcome by the provision of HRT under medical supervision. Specialists agree that the benefits of such therapy far outweigh the risks, but some members of the medical profession are yet to be convinced. In the mid 90s, it is important that research into new forms of treatment continues, but at the same time up-to-date information needs to be disseminated to all health care professionals and to women themselves, if full advantage is to be taken of the golden opportunity that HRT brings.

Malcolm Whitehead, Consultant Gynaecologist, Kings College Hospital, London

Appendix 3

Updating on latest HRT research

The Uterine Cancer Controversy

With each new edition of *No Change* Appendix 3 will be used to update information to give the very latest research findings relating to HRT. Medicine is a dynamic area in which situations are never static and HRT is no exception. It is my job to keep abreast of any changing views and to see that information is disseminated both in this book and in the press, so that both women and their doctors can properly assess the balance of risk and benefit.

Recent developments have largely concerned the uterine cancer scare, which emanated from America shortly after *No Change* was published in June 1975. British research happily has now resolved the problem, but in December 1975 there was considerable public concern following sensational press reports of studies published in the *New England Journal of Medicine* suggesting a 4.5 to 7.5 per cent increase in the risk of uterine cancer in women on long-term oestrogen therapy.

With an estimated ten million women on oestrogen replacement in the US, the Federal Drug Administration ordered an immediate enquiry, without even waiting to verify the findings of their interpretation. This rather precipitate step only added to the panic. In this country after our doctors had studied the American findings, there was only the merest hiccup in the steady ingestion of HRT into our medical system. The British view was that these retrospective studies were very open to criticism, and meanwhile their own ongoing prospective work would soon yield more reliable information.

Their man criticisms of the American work was that in most cases no account was taken of dosage or regimen (whether oestrogen was administered continuously or cyclically or whether a progestogen was added). also the selection of patients and controls was badly matched with no allowance made for such complicating factors as diabetes, obesity, parity (the number of children), etc., all known to also affect uterine cancer risks.

The most unfortunate matching applied to the largest study of all, that carried out by Dr Donald C. Smith in Seattle. He used as controls women also taken from the cancer registries but with other forms of gynaecological cancer, including a high percentage with cancer of the cervix. Now this form of cancer is traditionally associated with the lower socio-economic group, the very women in America least likely to be on HRT where it has to be paid for. In strong contrast uterine cancer is traditionally associated with the higher socio-economic group, obviously the very women *most* likely to be on HRT. Dr Smith very honestly pointed out in his paper that this fact could have inflated his figures, but his reservation was never reported in the press. There was also the very obvious fact that women on oestrogen get extra supervision, so that if they have cancer it is likely to be found early and make its way into the cancer registries.

This was very much borne out when I spoke to Dr Smith himself over the telephone in preparing an article for *World Medicine*.[1] He was frank enough to yield me the actual cancer category and distribution figures, never published until then, and even now not fully publicized in the US. They showed that of the 153 women in his study with uterine cancer found to be on oestrogen, 145 (95 per cent) were in categories 0 or 1.

Stage 1 is very early, invariably curable cancer and Stage 0 is not normally included in cancer statistics at all. Dr Smith himself made the point that the stages will usually regress in cyclic hormone therapy under the influence of oestrogen withdrawal and even more under the influence of progestogen, used in the combined form of HRT already mentioned in this book and also employed to actually treat this condition.

So only 5 per cent of oestrogen-treated women had serious cancer, with none at all in Stage 4 (deep invasive). But for women *not* on oestrogen it was a different story. Dr Smith's figures showed a total of forty-two out of the 164 non-oestrogen users (25 per cent) with serious cancer and seven of them in stage 4. So many experts argued that far from causing cancer HRT merely caused it to show up early, and certainly the five-year mortality figures for this study now available bear this out – only 7 per cent for women who had been on oestrogen but 37 per cent for those who had not. John Studd is convinced this points both to early diagnosis but also perhaps to hefty over-diagnosis by American doctors in interpreting border-line cases as cancer. This is understandable under a system where doctors go in constant fear of crippling litigation, a factor which may also account for the large numbers of unnecessary hysterectomies known to be performed in the US.

But with all that said, the American findings had too much significance to be ignored. Fortunately British research, particularly in the Chelsea, King's and Birmingham Menopause Clinics, was already tackling the problem. They were not relying on notoriously suspect retrospective studies, but on actual ongoing work, with endometrial biopsies carried out on all women both before and after starting HRT at their clinics, and comparing results on differing regimes of treatment.

The results did support the contention that there was some increased risk, but this was found to apply mainly to high-dose oestrogen and only to this when it was used without the protective action of progestogen (the synthetic version of progesterone taken by mouth). It was clear from the report given by Professor Stuart Campbell at the special Schering Workshop held at Sussex University in October 1977,[2] which I attended and reported in *Modern Medicine*,[3] that despite the cyclic system of three weeks on and one week off, a number of women failed to achieve the vital shedding required on oestrogen alone and there could be a build-up of lining over several cycles to give an abnormal thickening (hyperplasia). The incidence fell on lower-dose oestrogen, but was not entirely eliminated until a progestogen was added. In just a very few cancer-prone women hyperplasia may proceed toward malignancy if unchecked.

Another important factor reported by Dr Malcolm Whitehead, Senior Lecturer at King's College, emerged at the same meeting. He showed that presence or absence of breakthrough bleeding or withdrawal bleeding could not be considered a reliable indicator of either risk or safety. The studies showed hyperplasia could occur in the presence or absence of vaginal bleeding, and equally breakthrough bleeding could still occur in patients who proved to have perfectly normal endometrium.[4]

Since those first important studies another even more revealing series has been reported, this time carried out jointly by Birmingham and King's. These results, summarized by David Sturdee and his team,[5] confirmed that simple hyperplasia can be anticipated as a logical result of oestrogen stimulation, but again confirmed that use of a progestogen gave virtually complete protection. This second study, however, came up with a new and vital bit of information. It was found that ten days on a progestogen (in this case Norithesterone), with an overall dosage of only 15 mg over the period, gave better protection than five days with a higher dosage amounting to 25 mg in all. *So it is duration not dosage of the progestogen which is the vital protective factor.*

This should not be too surprising when one considers that this combined therapy is simulating nature's own method, and in the natural cycle progesterone comes into play in the second half of each cycle for between ten to fourteen days alongside oestrogen. If conception does not take place, as already explained earlier in the book, the levels of both hormones drop, allowing the lining that has built up to flow away, and the progestogen ensures this shedding is complete.

It is reassuring to know that in all cases of hyperplasia in these studies (and even in the very few cases of early uterine cancer) treatment with a progestogen achieved an effective cure.

The anti-HRT tide in America which temporarily ran so strong has reportedly turned, considerably helped by results of this British research. Meanwhile work by Dr Gambrell in the USAF Medical Centre at Lakeland, Texas,[6] parallels the British work but on an even larger scale. In a study of 2300 women with intact uteri (with wombs intact) 1060 were given oestrogen alone and five cases of uterine cancer were detected giving an incidence of 4.7 per 1000, a result in line with lowest findings of the original American studies. But with 1240 women treated with oestrogen and a progestogen, there was only one case of endometrial cancer, equivalent to only 0.8 per 1000. Dr Gambrell points out that this is less than in his own control sample of untreated menopausal women attending the same clinic, and also less than the known spontaneous incidence of this disease. As in the British study, reversion of hyperplasia was achieved in all cases treated with progestogen.

So at last firm guidelines can be laid down both for doctor and patient. The lowest dosage of oestrogen should be used to effectively relieve symptoms and ten to twelve days' course of progestogen added each cycle. With this method it is not even necessary for the woman to stop oestrogen therapy each month, if she is one of those who find symptoms return even in one week off medication.

Most gynaecologists are now so confident about the protective action of progestogen in HRT, that they no longer feel the safeguard of a regular endometrial check every two years is necessary.

The drug companies have played their part very fully in all this, firstly by financing the research which has established the vital role of progestogen, and secondly by producing 'combined packs' with progestogen built in to simplify prescribing and usage. But any doctor who prefers can still prescribe a suitable progestogen to be taken for ten or twelve days alongside the oestrogen of his choice.

The woman must play her part by accepting the light withdrawal bleed this system involves. The recent studies showed that 90 per cent of patients were quite happy about this, once the reasons were fully explained.

In 1996 there is no excuse for doctors failing to prescribe one of the proven and safe forms of HRT and encouraging patients to stay on treatment for the necessary minimum of five years to ensure the important bonus of adequate skeletal and cardio-vascular protection.

A European Survey

The findings of a very large study carried out by the International Health Foundation among physicians and women in the UK, France and West Germany, published in 1995, revealed interesting differences in information levels on HRT and osteoporosis across the three countries.

Eighty-three per cent of women questioned in this country were aware of the link between the menopause and risk of brittle bones, as opposed to only 70 per cent of French women and 41 per cent of German. This almost certainly reflects the excellent work of the NOS here in achieving such a high profile for osteoporosis in the press, TV and radio: 81 per cent of British women said they had got their information from the media or books, as against only 8 per cent from their doctors. This last figure contrasted with 50 per cent informed by doctors in France and 30 per cent in Germany.

Resumption of menstrual bleeding was found to exert the most influence in dissuading women from starting treatment or in coming off too soon. Doctors themselves estimated the proportions of women treated who would stay on HRT long enough to effectively prevent osteoporosis as only 38 per cent in France, 50 per cent in Germany and 40 per cent in Britain. This figure seems to represent an over-optimistic estimate by doctors where this country is concerned, but clearly it is not only here that the message of long-term benefit needs to be emphasized.

Prevention of Colon Cancer

1996 saw the publication in the *Journal of the National Cancer Institute* of a study involving many thousands of women in the US suggesting a link between the use of oestrogen in HRT and a reduction in the death rate from bowel cancer. The link was still there even after women had stopped using HRT and the Institute is calling for more studies to be done.

Osteoporosis

Teeth It has recently been emphasized that loss of bone produces osteoporotic changes not only in the spine and limbs but also in the jaws. This causes teeth to work loose, allowing food to become trapped around them and leading to gum recession. An American study reported in the British medical publication, *General Practitioner*, looked at the teeth of 6000 retired women and found that those taking HRT were only half as likely to have lost their teeth, and only 20 per cent as liable to need dentures.

The Role of Exercise Studies continue to confirm the

vital importance of exercise in building and maintaining strong bones. This was shown to apply to the young as well as the old, with a recent study of 1359 children aged seven to eleven finding that exercise increased bone mineral density, while no similar link was found between a high-calcium diet and stronger bones. In the *Journal of Epidemiology and Community Health*, the point was made that in order to lay down calcium, bones need to be stressed by exercise. Hopefully plans for more compulsory games and gym within the school curriculum may help.

A Blood Test to Identify Osteoporosis Risk   There have long been hopes of a blood test which could identify people at high risk of osteoporosis. In 1995 doctors at St Thomas's Hospital were able to announce development of just such a test. Rooted in the latest genetic technology it relies on the recent discovery of a gene on chromosome 12 that has been shown to affect bone density in later life. Known as the vitamin D receptor gene, it occurs in three different forms, with people carrying the 'at risk' variant having lower bone density and a 50 per cent higher risk of fractures.

Accordingly, the team at St Thomas's carried out a three-year study of 95 pairs of identical twins and 87 pairs of non-identical twins. Their findings have now established that identical twins sharing similar genes also share similar bone densities. In contrast, the non-identical twins, who did not have the same variant of the vitamin D receptor gene, had large differences in bone density. It is believed the gene works by controlling the body's use of vitamin D and thus absorption of calcium.

On this premise, work is continuing with further pairs of twins to test just how effective vitamin D supplements may be in actually preventing bone loss. It is pointed out, however, that even if this trial proves successful, it will not obviate the value of HRT at the menopause to counter the accelerated bone loss that follows ovarian failure.

The blood test will also not identify low bone density and brittle bone risk due to – *non*-genetic causes such as inadequate diet, lack of exercise, use of steroids, heavy smoking or premature natural or surgical menopause. Some modification is still required before the new test can be made generally available, but eventually it should offer a welcome new weapon in the fight against brittle bones and consequent fractures.

A Urine Test for Osteoporosis Risk Advances are coming thick and fast in the battle against this disease, responsible currently for more than 100,000 hip fractures a year in Britain. In 1995 yet another simple test was announced, this time costing only £10. Developed by the Rowett Research Institute in Aberdeen and called the Pyrilinks-D test, it uses a urine sample to pick up information which can detect the rate at which bone is being lost. If further validated such a test will have immense value in identifying fast bone-losers and persuading them to go on HRT and to stay on for at least five years. It can also monitor treatment and demonstrate how HRT has reduced bone loss, providing an incentive to continue treatment. It could offer a cheap screening system to pinpoint those women who would benefit from bone density scanning to check for potential fracture sites.

Medical references

The references are presented in the following order: the name or names of the author or authors: the year of publication; the title of the journal; the volume number; further volume reference number (if applicable); page number.

Chapter 4

1. Gordan, C.S. (1973), *American Family Physician* 8, 6, 74.
2. Nordin, B.E.C., Gallagher, J.C. (1972), *The Lancet* 1, 503.
   Nordin, B.E.C., Gallagher, J.C. (1972), *Clinical Endocrinology* 1, 57.
   Nordin, B.E.C., Gallagher, J.C. (1973), *Pulse* 26, 10, 24.
   Nordin, B.E.C. (1971), *British Medical Journal* 1, 571.
3. Aitken, J.M., Hart, D.M., Lindsay, R. (1973), *British Medical Journal* 3, 515.
4. Atkins, D., Zanelli, J.M., Peacock, M., Nordin, B.E.C. (1972), *Journal of Endocrinology* 54, 107.
5. Christiansen, C., Christiansen, M.S., et al (1981) *The Lancet* 1, 1038–1040.
   Munk-Jenson, et al (1988), *British Medical Journal* 296, 1150–1152.
   Selby, P.L., et al (1985), *Clinical Science* 69, 265–271.
6. Studd, J.W.W., Fogelman, I. (1990), *American Journal of Obstetrics and Gynecology* 163: No. 5, 1474–1479.
7. Wilson, R.A., Wilson, Thelma A. (1963), *Journal of American Geriatric Society* 11, 347.
   Wilson, R.A. (1964), *Chicago Medical Journal* 67, 193.
8. Villalodid, L.S., Buenaluz, L., Iledan, A. (1973), *Current Medical Research and Opinion* 1, 10, 577.
9. Oliver, M.F., Boyd, G.S. (1959), *The Lancet* 1, 690.
10. Stampfer, M.K., Willett, W.C., et al (1985), *New England*

Medical Journal 318, 1044–1049.
Kaplan, N.M. (1985), *Journal of Reproductive Medicine* 30, 910, 802–804.
Henderson, B.E., et al (1986), *American Journal of Obstetrics* 154, 1181–1186.
Colditz, G.A., et al (1987), *New England Journal of Medicine* 416, 1105–1110.
11. McBride, W.G. (1967), *Post-Graduate Medical Journal* 43, 55.
12. Kantor, H.I., Michael, C.M., Shore, H., Ludvigson, H.W. (1968), *American Journal of Obstetrics and Gynecology* 101, 5, 568.
Kantor, H.I., Michael, C.M., Shore, H. (1973), *American Journal of Obstetrics and Gynecology* 116, 1, 115.
Michael, C.M., Kantor, H.I., Shore, H. (1970), *Journal of Gerontology* 25, 4, 337.
13. Paganini-Hill, A., Buckwalter, J.G., et al (1993), *Society for Neuroscience Abstracts* 19, 1046.
Mestel, R. (1993), *New Scientist* No. 1900: 10.

Chapter 5
1. Gordan, C.S. (1973), *American Family Physician* 8, 6, 74; (1963–64), *Yearbook of Cancer*.
2. Bakke, J.L. (1963), *Western Journal of Surgery, Obstetrics and Gynecology* 71, 241.
3. Burch, J.C., Byrd, B.F. (1971), *Annals of Surgery* 174, 3, 414.
Burch, J.C., Byrd, B.F., Vaughan, W.K. (1974), *American Journal of Obstetrics and Gynecology* 118, 6, 778.
4. Hunt, K., Vessey, M., McPherson, K., Coleman, M. (1987, *British Journal of Obstetrics and Gynaecology* 94, 621–635.
5. Bland, K.I. (1979), *Proceedings of International Symposium on Menopause*, Rome (MTP Press).
6. Gambrell, R.D. (1983), *Obstetrics and Gynaecology* 662, 438–443.
Gambrell, R.D. (1986), *International Journal of Fertility* 31, 112–122.
7. Sturdee, D.W., Wade-Evans, Studd, J. (1977), *British Journal of Obstetrics and Gynaecology* 84, 193–195.
Campbell, S., et al (1978) *Postgraduate Medical Journal* 54, 59–64.

Sturdee, D.W., Paterson, M.E., et al (1978), *British Medical Journal* 1, 1575–1577.

8. Nicol, T., Builbey, D., et al (1964), *Journal of Endocrinology* 30, 277.
   Nicol, T., Vernon-Roberts, B. (1965), *Journal of Endocrinology* 33, 365.

9. Newcomb, et al (1995), *Am. J. Epidem.* 142, 788–795.

Chapter 6

1. Moore, B., Magnani, H., Studd, J. (1974), *Journal of Obstetrics and Gynaecology of the British Commonwealth* 81, 12, 1005.

2. Bolton, C.H., Hampton, J.R., Mitchell, J.R.A. (1968), *The Lancet* 2, 315.

3. Stevenson, J.C., Whitehead, M.I. (1982), *British Medical Journal*, 285, 586–587.

4. Lacassagne, A. (1932), Comptes Rendus Académie des Sciences 195, 630.

5. Cutler, S.J., Connolly, R.R. (1969), *Cancer* 23, 767.

6. Herbst, A.C., Robboy, S.I., et al (1974), *American Journal of Obstetrics and Gynecology* 119, 5, 713.

7. Sturdee, D.W., Studd, J., et al (1977), *British Journal of Obstetrics and Gynaecology* 84, 193–195.
   Sturdee, D.W., Patterson, M.E., et al (1978), *British Medical Journal* 1, 1575–1577.

Chapter 9

1. Marmorston, J., Magidson, O., Lewis, J.J., Mehl, J., Moore, F.J., Bernstein, J. (1958), *The New England Journal of Medicine* 258, 12, 583.

2. Rauramo, L., Punnonen, R. (1972), *Frontiers of Hormone Research* 2, 48.

3. Savvas, M., Studd, J., et al (1993), *British Journal of Obstetrics and Gynaecology* 100, 154–156.
   Holland, E.F.N., Studd, J., et al (1994), *Journal of Obstetrics and Gynaecology* 83: No. 2, 180–183.

4. Lauritzen, C. (1972), *Frontiers of Hormone Research* 2, 2.

5. Notelovitz, M. (1975), *South African Medical Journal* 49, 2251–2255.

6. Barrett-Connor, E., et al (1979), *Journal of American Medicine Association* 241, 2167–2170.

7. Kaye, S.A., et al (1990), *International Journal of Obesity* 14, 583–591.
8. Orimo, H., et al (1970), *Journal of American Geriatric Society* 18, 1, 11.
9. Jaszmann, L. (1972), *Frontiers of Hormone Research* 2, 22.
10. Alyward, M. (1973), *RCS Int. Research Com. Systems* (373–7), 3, 5, 11.
11. Richards, D.M. (1973), *The Lancet* 11, 430.
12. Siddle, N., Whitehead, M. (1986), *Fertility and Sterility* 47, 95–100.
13. Quinn, A.J., Barrett, T., et al (1994), Journal of Obstetrics and Gynaecology 14, 103–107.
14. Oldenhave, A., et al (1993), *American Journal of Obstetrics and Gynecology* 168, 765–771.
15. Panel on Ovarian Conservation v Extirpation (1974), *The Menopausal Syndrome* (Ed. R. Greenblatt) p. 186 (Medcom Press, NY).

Chapter 11
1. Moore, B., Gustafson, R., Studd, J.W. (1974), *Journal of Obstetrics and Gynaecology of the British Commonwealth* 81, 12, 1005.
2. Lane, G., Siddle, N.C., Whitehead, M.T., et al (1986), *British Journal of Obstetrics and Gynaecology* 93, 55–62.
3. Lauritzen, C. (1972), *Frontiers of Hormone Research* 2, 2.

Chapter 12
1. Greenblatt, R.B. (1950), *Clinical Endocrinology* 10, 1547.
   Greenblatt, R.B. (1965), *New England Journal of Medicine* 272, 305.
   Greenblatt, R.B. (1972), *Clinician-Med. Gynaecology* p. 30.
   Greenblatt, R.B. (1972), *Medical Counterpart* 4, 15.
   Greenblatt, R.B. (1974), *The Menopausal Syndrome* (p. 95–102 and 222–230).
2. Studd, J., Brincat, M., Magos, A., Cadaza, L.D., et al (1984), *The Lancet* 1, 16–18.
   Studd, J., Savvas, M., et al (1992) *British Journal of*

Obstetrics and Gynaecology 99, 757–760.
Studd, J., Savvas, M., et al (1993), *British Journal of Obstetrics and Gynaecology* 100, 154–156.
3. Hunter, D.J.S., Julier, D., Bonnar, J. (1974), *20th British Congress of Obstetrics and Gynaecology*, Scientific Programme, p. 67.
Hunter, D.J.S., Akande, E.O., Carr, P., Stallworthy, J. (1973), *Journal of Obstetrics and Gynaecology of the British Commonwealth* 80, 827.

Appendix 3
1. Smith, D.C. (1975), *New England Journal of Medicine* 293, 1164.
2. Campbell, S., et al (1978), *Postgraduate Medical Journal* 54 (Suppl. 2): 59–64.
3. Cooper, W. (1978), *Modern Medicine*, January.
4. Whitehead, M. (1978), Maturitas 1, 87–98.
5. Sturdee, D.W., Paterson, M.E.L., et al (1978), *British Medical Journal* 1, 1575–1577.

Other medical papers relating to HRT

Osteoporosis

1. Conference report. Consensus development conference: prophylaxis and treatment of osteoporosis.
   Br. Med. J. (1987); *285*: 914–916.

   – excellent summary of the current thinking about post-menopausal osteoporosis and its treatment produced by the 1987 meeting of the European Formulation for Osteoporosis and Bone Disease.

2. Prediction of rapid bone loss in post-menopausal women. Christiansen, C. *et al.* (1987); The Lancet, May 16: 1105–1108.

   – describes the work of one of the world's foremost experts on osteoporosis regarding tests designed to predict those post-menopausal women who lose bone rapidly and who would therefore be at most risk of fractures.

3. Prevention of post-menopausal bone loss – Effects of alternative administration forms of oestrogens, alternative gestogens and calcium addition.
   Riss, B.J. & Christiansen, C. (1987); NucCompact, *18*: 24–28.

   – study of alternative forms of HRT and their effectiveness in preventing bone loss.

4. Managing osteoporosis: Current trends, future possibilities.
   Lindsay, R. (1987); Geriatrics, *42* (3): 35–40.

   – review paper by the top expert on osteoporosis.

5. A Clinic for the prevention of Osteoporosis in general

practice.
Coope, J., Roberts, D. (1990), *British Journal of General Practice* 40, No. 336.

6. *New techniques in Metabolic Bone Disease.*
Ed. Stevenson, J.C. (1990), Wright, London.

Endometrial Cancer

1. Endometrial disease after treatment with oestrogens and progestogens in the climacteric.
Paterson, M.E.L. *et al.* (1980); Br. Med. J. *280*: 822–824.

   – study investigating the number of days progestogen per cycle necessary to prevent the development of endometrial cancer.

2. Prevention of endometrial abnormalities.
Whitehead, M.I. (1986); Acta. Obstet. Gynecol. Scand. Suppl. 134: 81–91.

   – review on this subject by a top UK expert.

Breast Cancer

1. Hormone replacement therapy and breast cancer.
Gambrell, R.D. (1987); Maturitas, *9*: 123–133.

   – excellent up-to-date review on the current situation from the world's leading authority on HRT and breast cancer.

2. Non-contraceptive oestrogen use and the risk of breast cancer.
Kaufman, D.W. *et al.* (1984); J.A.M.A. *252* (1): 63–67.

   – large case-control study suggesting that HRT does not increase the risk of breast cancer.

3. The risk of breast cancer in post-menopausal women who have used oestrogen replacement therapy.
Wingo, P.A. *et al.* (1987); J.A.M.A. *257* (2): 209–215.

   – another large case-control study showing no appreciable increase in breast cancer risk with increasing HRT duration or latency, even for durations and latencies of 20 years or longer.

Cardio-vascular Disease

1. Non-contraceptive oestrogen use and cardio-vascular

disease.

Bush, T.L. & Barrett-Connor, E. (1985); Epidemiologic Reviews, 7: 80–104.

– excellent review of the biological effects of HRT on various blood parameters as well as a large number of clinical studies.

2. Estrogen replacement therapy: Effect on blood pressure and other cardio-vascular risk factors.
Kaplan, N.M. (1985); J. Reprod. Med. *30* (10): 802–804.

– short review discussing the cardio-protective effect of HRT.

3. Estrogen use and cardio-vascular disease.
Henderson, B.E. *et al.* (1986); Am. J. Obstet. Gynecol. *154*: 1181–1186.

– review of many case-control and cohort studies which demonstrate a cardio-protective effect for HRT.

4. Menopause and the risk of coronary heart disease in women.
Colditz, G.A. *et al.* (1987); N. Eng. J. Med. *316*: 1105–1110.

– recent study which demonstrated that HRT prevented the increase in the risk of coronary heart disease in oophorectomized women.

General

1. Estrogen replacement therapy: Current thinking and practice.
De Fazio, J. & Speroff, L. (1985); Geriatrics, *40* (11): 32–48.

– excellent review on HRT.

2. Oestrogen deficiency: Causes, consequences and management.
Padwick, M. & Whitehead, M. (1985); Update, August: 275–284.

– review by two top UKexperts.

3. A review of study findings of the risks and benefits of oestrogen therapy in the female climacteric.
Rauramo, L. (1986); Maturitas, *8*: 177–187.

– a review which concludes that the relative risk of death in oestrogen users aged over 40 is markedly lower than in non-users.

4. *Hormone Replacement Therapy* (1990), Coope, J., RCGP, London.

5. *The Menopause* (1988), Studd, W.W., Whitehead, M.A., Blackwell Scientific.

Advisory and support bodies

Women's Health Concern
93–99 Upper Richard Road, London SW15 2TB
Tel: 0181–780–3916
Helpline: 0181–780–3007

Under the name of Women's Health Care, this was the first organization dedicated to educating and advising women about the menopause and the proper use of Hormone Replacement Therapy. Started in 1972 by Joan Jenkins it became legally constituted in 1977 with a Medical Advisory Board. In 1978 under the new name of Women's Health Concern it became a registered charity.

Joan Jenkins continued as Founder-Coordinator and Dr Gerald Sywer, the eminent Consultant Endocrinologist, served as Founder Chairman until shortly before his death in September 1995. This honorary post has now been filled by Dr John Stevenson, another well known Consultant Endocrinologist and currently Head of the Wynn Institute for Metabolic Research in London.

The work of WHC has expanded to cover a whole range of gynaecological problems, and special leaflets are free to anyone who writes enclosing an SAE. In recent years the work of advancing health education among women has been extended into professional areas, with the organization of Medical Symposia, special nurses' study days and one-week courses for nurse counsellors.

WHC funds re donated by companies, banks, trusts, other organizations and individuals, with the workload also recognized since 1980 by a Section 64 Grant from the Department of Health.

Anyone needing practical help or advice can write (with SAE) to the above address or ring the Helpline number.

The National Osteoporosis Society (NOS)
PO Box 10, Radstock, Bath, BA3 3YB
Tel: 01761–471771

Established in 1986, the National Osteoporosis Society is the only charity dedicated exclusively to improving the diagnosis, treatment and prevention of osteoporosis. NOS Founder Chairman, Dr Allan Dixon, helped set up the charity, in his own words to 'harness people power, to influence politicians and doctors regarding the magnitude of the national osteoporosis problem so that something would be done about it.' The Society's current Chairman is Consultant Gynaecologist Mr John Studd, and the charity has its own board of medical advisors who represent all the different disciplines involved in osteoporosis.

The Society is very active in educating the general public as to how osteoporosis can be prevented. There is no cure for osteoporosis so early action to develop and then maintain a strong skeleton throughout life is essential. The healthy bones message is communicated through media campaigns, public meetings, talks to women's groups, a children's education campaign, the important work of local support groups and regular newsletters to NOS members. The Society receives each year approximately 250,000 requests for advice and information via telephone calls and letters. All receive an individual reply and an S.A.E. would help with this.

The NOS also works closely with healthcare professionals to keep them informed of developments in the management of osteoporosis. 1000 professional members are kept up-to-date via the Society's journal, *Osteoporosis Review*, and the Society is now running nurse study days to inform nurses of how they can improve osteoporosis care. In 1993 the Society sent its *Menopause and Osteoporosis Therapy* pack to every GP surgery in the UK to help doctors identify people at risk of the disease, and to ensure that established sufferers receive appropriate treatment.

A major step forward in improving osteoporosis care was achieved in 1995 with the publication of a Government Report on the disease. The NOS was represented on the panel of experts who drew up the Report's recommendations, which called for an effective osteoporosis service to be set up by each health authority. The Society is now campaigning for the Report's recommendations to be implemented in every health district.

Sadly the number of fractures are continuing to rise at a rate of 10 per cent per year. Research is desperately needed to understand why so many more people are at risk of the disease. The NOS is now actively fundraising for research into osteoporosis to try to ensure that future generations do not suffer from the devastating disease. When The Great British Bone Appeal was launched in 1989 with a target of £1 million to fund and expand their work, the first donations received were from The Queen and The Queen Mother. Annual Membership fees are £15 for Non sufferers, £10 for Sufferers, £8 for Junior Supporters and £20 for Healthcare Professionals.

The Amarant Trust
11–13 Charterhouse Buildings, London EC1M 7AN
Tel: 0171–490–1644
Menopause and HRT Helplines: 0891–60620

Amarant was a mythical, never-fading flower, which was a symbol of immortality and enduring beauty to the Greeks. It was chosen as an appropriate name for a charitable trust set up in 1986, by Malcolm Whitehead, Consultant Gynaecologist at King's College Hospital, who has been an outstanding pioneer of HRT in Britain. One of the aims of Amarant includes raising funds to enable the valuable HRT and menopause research, carried out at King's College Hospital, to be continued and expanded.

In addition, however, Amarant aims to promote a better understanding of the menopause and the biological changes that occur in women from their mid-forties as hormone levels decline. At the same time, it sets out to alert women to the existence of HRT, which by replacing the missing hormones can combat these changes, restore the quality of life, eliminate menopause symptoms and, in particular, prevent the increased bone loss that can lead to post-menopausal osteoporosis.

At medical level this is done by a team of King's College

specialists through post-graduate meetings and special study days for GPs (invariably over-subscribed). These offer the opportunity for the latest information on HRT techniques and research to be diseminated and for any prescribing or diagnostic problems to be discussed. This medical education work is now being extended to other health professionals.

At lay level, information and advice is available via leaflets, booklets, video and audio tapes as well as through ten special telephone helplines. Personal advice, assessment and treatment is also available at the Amarant Centre, a self- or GP-referral clinic manned by King's College doctors and sited at London's Churchill Clinic. Other additional services can also be obtained such as cervical smears, thyroid function tests, mammograms, etc. This is the first of many such self-referral centres planned as more resources become available.

A new and important facet of Amarant work, however, concerns the setting up of Amarant groups – these local support groups, now proliferating across the country, are designed to boost morale and increase understanding through exchange of information and experience. Anyone interested in joining such a group (or starting one in their own area) can apply to Amarant for information.

Although the work of the Amarant Trust is assisted by a modest DHSS grant, it relies for income mainly on modest DOH grant, it relies for income mainly on the £20 annual fee from Friends of the Trust, donations from other private individuals and from companies, and money made on the sale of Amarant tapes, books and telephone helplines. Booklets and regular newsletters are mailed free to Friends, who can also take advantage of a telephone advice line manned by a specialist menopause counsellor. Full details can be obtained from The Amarant Trust at the above address.

Family Planning Association
Family Planning National Office, 27–35 Mortimer Street, London W1N 7RJ
Tel: 0171–636–7866

The FPA has served women for so long and so well that their work has often been taken for granted. Since 1974, however, their clinics have been gradually handed over to the NHS to be run by local authorities. Unfortunately, this means that neither provision of HRT nor referral facilities can be guaranteed. However, the FPA are continuing their work on health research and education and this includes advising on the menopause, HRT, and how and where to obtain this treatment in various areas of the country. For information contact their national office.

Cystitis Counselling
Angela Kilmartin, 75 Mortimer Road, London N1
Tel: 0171–249–8664

Although the U and I Club, set up by Angela Kilmartin was closed down some years ago, she is still lecturing and also does personal counselling from the above address.

List of menopause and HRT clinics

Key: § National Health Service (NHS)
Private
* Charge made (on a non-profitmaking basis)

Aberdeen: § Dr Anderson, Aberdeen Royal Infirmary Foresthill, Aberdeen AB9 QZB (01225 681818)
also: § Dr Jandial, Menopause Clinic, Aberdeen Royal Infirmary Foresthill, Aberdeen AB9 QZN (01224 681818)
Airdrie: § Mrs A. White, Health Department, Adam Avenue, Airdrie (0123 69229)
Ashford: § Dr Stewart, Menopause Clinic, William Harvey Hospital, Kennington Road, Ashford, Kent (01233 633331)
also: § Mr P. Saunders, Gynaecology Dept., Ashford Hospital, London Road, Ashford (01784 251188)
Bangor: # Greenhouse, Trevelyan Terrace, Bangor (01248 352176)
Barnsley: § Dr Wunna, Menopause Advisory Clinic, Family Planning Clinic, Queens Road, Barnsley, South Yorkshire (01226 730000)
Barrow-in-Furness: § Dr Jill Tattersall, Well Woman Clinic, Atinson Road, Barrow-in-Furness, Cumbria (01229 27212)
Basingstoke: § Mrs Hemington, Fairfield's Clinic, Fairfield's Road, Basingstoke RG24 (01256 26980)
Beckenham: § Mr J. McQueen, Gynaecology Department, Beckenham Hospital, 379 Croydon Road, Beckenham, Kent (0181 650 0125)
Belfast: § Mr J. Houston, Samaritan Hospital, Lisburn Road, Belfast (01232 332300)
also: § Prof. Thompson, HRT Clinic, Belfast Maternity

Hospital, Grosvenor Road, Belfast BT12 6BA (01232 240503)

Birmingham: # Miss D. Gray, St Mary's Road, Harborne, Birmingham B17 0HA (0121 427 6525)

also: § Dr Gillian Stuart, Menopause Clinic, Maternity Hospital, Queen Elizabeth Medical Centre, Birmingham B15 2TG (0121 472 1377)

also: § Dr Gillian Stuart, Birmingham and Midland Hospital for Women, Showall Green Lane, Sparkhill, Birmingham B11 (0121 722 1101)

also: # Dr Gillian Stuart, AMI Priory Hospital, 22 Priory Road, Edgbaston, Birmingham B5 7UG (0121 440 6611)

also: # Dr Gillian Stuart, The Edgbaston Nuffield Hospital, 22 Somerset Road, Edgbaston, Birmingham B15 2QD (0121 456 2000)

also: # Mr J. Jordan, 20 Church Road, Edgbaston, Birmingham B15 (0121 454 2345)

also: § Dr P. Plant, Menopause Clinic, 5 York Road, Birmingham B16 9HH (0121 454 8236)

also: § Dr P. Plant, Menopause Counselling, St Patrick's Family Planning Clinic, Highgate Street, Birmingham B12 0YA (0121 440 2422)

also: § Dr Mushin, Soho Health Centre, Louise Road, Handsworth, Birmingham (0121 523 9231)

also: § Dr Threlfall, Warren Farm Health Centre, Warren Farm Road, Kingstanding, Birmingham (0121 373 1740)

also: § Dr Threlfall and Dr Ahamed, Aston Health Centre, Trinity Road, Aston, Birmingham (0121 328 7900)

also: § Dr Thake, Annie Wood Resource Centre, Alma Way, Lozells, Birmingham (0121 554 7137/3155)

also: * Midland Clinic, 5 York Road, Birmingham B16 9HX (0121 454 8236)

Blackrock: § Dr M. Short and Dr G. Kearus, Women's Medical Centre, 34 Main Street, Blackrock (0110 3531 884943)

Bournemouth: # Dr Susan Parker, 2 Clarendon Road, Westbourne, Dorset BH4 8AH (01202 764803)

Brighton: § Mr Beard, Family Planning Clinic, Morely Street, Brighton, East Sussex BN2 2RA (01273 693600)

also: § Mr Malville, Royal Sussex Hospital, Eastern Road, Brighton, Sussex BN2 5BE (01273 696955)

also: § Mr R. Bradley, Gynaecology Department, Brighton

General Hospital, Elm Grove, Brighton BN3 3RX
(01272 696011)

Braintree: § St Michael's Day Hospital, Rayne Road, Braintree (01245 261749)

Bristol: # Dr Ruth Coles, Richmond Hill Clinic, 25 Denmark Street, Bristol BS1 5DQ (01272 292183)

Buckingham: § Dr Brown, Family Planning Clinic, Buckingham Hospital, Buckingham Town, Bucks MK18 1NU (01280 813243)

Burton-on-Trent: § Dr Naomi Spencer, Burton District Hospital, Belvedere Road, Burton-on-Trent, Staffordshire DE13 0RB (01283 66333)

also: § Dr Naomi Spencer, Bridge Street Surgery, 23 Bridge Street, Burton-on-Trent (01283 63451)

Cambridge: § The Menopause Clinic, Maternity Hospital, Dept. of Obstetrics, Cambridge CB2 5W (01223 336875)

Cheadle: * Dr Y. Steadman, Lifestyle Dept., AMI Alexandra Hospital, Mill Lane, Cheadle SK8 2PX (0161 428 3565)

Chelmsford: § The Health Clinic, Springfield Green, Essex (01245 261749)

Chester: § Mr John Williams, Family Planning Clinic, Maternity Unit, Countess of Chester Hospital, Liverpool Road, Chester (01244 365000)

Consett: § Mr Johnson, Menopause Clinic, Out-patients Department, Shotley Bridge General Hospital, Shotley Bridge, Consett, Co Durham BH8 0NB (01207 503456)

Crewe: # Amarant Centre at The South Cheshire Private Hospital, Leighton, Crewe VCW1 4QP (01270 500411)

Doncaster: § Health Centre, Crooksbroom Lane, Hatfield, Doncaster CN7 6JQ (01302 841373)

Dublin: * Rita Burtenshaw, Dublin Well Woman Centre, 73 Lower Lesson Street, Dublin 2 (610083/610086)

also: § Dr N. Cleary, Coombe Hospital, Dublin (537561)

also: # Ms H. Walsh, 59 Synge Street, Dublin 8 (780712)

also: # Dr Kearns, 5–7 Catbal Brugha Street, Dublin 1 (727726/723363)

also: # Dr M. Woods, Ailesbury Road, Dublin 4 (011 696894)

Edinburgh: § Dr J. Bancroft, Dean Terrace Centre, 18 Dean Terrace, Edinburgh EH4 1NL (0131 332 7941/0131 343 243)

also: § Mr White, Edinburgh Royal Infirmary, 39 Chalmers Street, Edinburgh (0131 229 2477)

Exeter: * Well Woman Clinic, Alice Vieland Clinic, Bull Meadow Road, Exeter (01392 72741)

Gateshead: Mr Silverstone, Queen Elizabeth Hospital, Gateshead, Tyne and Wear (0191 487 8989)

Glasgow: § Dr Helen McEwan, Glasgow Royal Infirmary, Castle Street, Glasgow G4 0SF (0141 552 3535)

also: § Dr David McKay Hart, Bone Metabolism Research Unit, Western Infirmary, Glasgow G11 6NT (0141 339 8822)

also: § Dr David McKay Hart, Stobhill Hospital, Balornock Road, Glasgow G21 (0141 558 0111)

also: § Dr E. Wilson, Family Planning Centre, 2 Claremont Terrace, Glasgow G3 (0141 332 9411)

also: § Miss Fraser (Mondays 7.30 to 9.00p.m.), Central Health Centre, North Carbrain Road, Cumbernauld, Glasgow G67 1BJ (01236 731771)

Grimsby: § Winn Davey, Well Woman Centre, Eleanor Street, Grimsby, South Humberside (01472 362098)

Hatfield: # Dr Brenda Bean, Medical Centre, Hatfield Polytechnic College, College Lane, Hatfield, Herts (01707 279444)

Havant: # Dr Sarah Randall, BUPA Hospital, Portsmouth, Bartons Road, Havant, Hants PO9 5NP (01705 454511)

also: § Dr Thomas, Menopausal Clinic, Havant Health Centre, Civic Centre Road, Havant PO9 2AZ (01705 455111)

High Wycombe: * Dr Chapman, The Wycombe Clinic, 6 Harlow Road, High Wycombe, Bucks HP13 6AA (01494 26666)

Hove: # Dr Jones, 32 Westbourne Villas, Hove, Sussex (01273 720217)

also: § Well Woman Clinic, Mortimer House, 12A Western Road, Hove, East Sussex (01273 774075)

Hull: § Prof. D. Prudie, Princess Royal Hospital, Salthouse Road, Hull (01482 701151)

also: * Well Woman Clinic, Central Clinic, 79 Beverely Road, Kingston-upon-Hull (014822 28888)

Keighley: § Dr D. Miles, Airedale General Hospital, Steeton, Keighley, West Yorkshire BD20 6TD (01535 52511 x 442)

Kendal: § Dr Daphne Lowe, Well Woman Clinic, Blackhall Road, Kendal, Cumbria (01935 727564)

Kenilworth: § Dr Felicity Smith, Menopause Advice Clinic, Kenilworth Clinic, Smalley Place, Kenilworth, Warwickshire (01926 52087)

Leeds: § Dr Mary Jones, Clarendon Wing, Leeds General Infirmary, Belmont Grove, Leeds LS2 9NS (01532 432799 x 3886)

Liverpool: § Mr R. Farquharson, Menopause Clinic, The Womens' Hospital, Catherine Street, Liverpool L8 7NJ (0151 709 1000)

also: # Mr R. G. Farquharson, 31 Rodney Street, Liverpool L1 9EH (0151 709 8522)

also: § Dr Carter, Cytology Department, Community Headquarters, Sefton General Hospital, Smithdown Road, Liverpool L15 2HE (0151 733 4020 x 2555)

also: # Mr H. Francis, 25 Britannia Pavilion, Albert Dock, Liverpool L3 (0151 709 3998)

London: § Mrs T.R. Varma, Consultant Gynaecologist, St George's Medical School and Hospital, Blackshaw Road, London SW17 (0181 672 1255)

also: * Dr Kouba, Marie Stopes Clinic, 108 Whitfield Street, London W1 (0171 388 0662/2585)

also: Dr Mary Griffin, PMT and Menopause Clinic, The London Hospital, Whitechapel, London E1 1B (0171 377 7000 x 2030)

also: § Dr Shamougan, Park Lane Clinic, 131 Park Lane, London N17 (0181 808 9094)

also: § Dr Nicholls, Crouch End Health Centre, 45 Middle Lane, London N8 (0181 341 2045)

also: § Dr Shamougan, Stuart Crescent Health Centre, 8 Stuart Crescent, London N22 (0181 889 4311)

also: # Mr N. Cullen, BUPA Screen Unit for Women, BUPA Medical Centre, Battle Bridge House, 300 Grays In Road, London WC1X 8DU (0171 837 6484 x 2304)

also: § Mr Ballard, Queen Mary's Hospital, Roehampton Lane, Roehampton, London SW15 5PN (0181 789 6611)

also: § Patrick Doody Clinic, Pelham Road, London SW19 (0181 685 9922)

also: * The Amarant Centre, 80 Lambeth Road, London SE1 7PW (0171 401 3855)

also: # Mr John Studd, 120 Harley Street, London W1N 1AG (0171 486 0497/7641) *also*: # Mr John Studd, Lister Hospital, Chelsea Bridge Road, London SW1 (0171 730 5433/3417)

also: § Mr John Studd, Chelsea and Westminster Hospital, 369 Fulham Road, London SW10 (0171 741 8000)

also: § Mr Malcolm Whitehead, Menopause Clinic, Queen Charlottes Hospital, Goldhawk Road, London W6 0XG (0181 740 3910)

also: § Mr Malcolm Whitehead, Menopause Clinic, King's College Hospital, Denmark Hill, London SE5 9RS (0181 733 0224)

also: # Dr G. Chodhury, 886 Garratt Lane, London SW17 (0181 648 3234)

also: § Mr P. Saunders, Menopause Clinic, Gynaecology Out-Patients Department, St Thomas Hospital, Lambeth Place Road, London SE1 (0171 928 9292 x 2533)

also: # Dr C. Mortimer, Osteoporosis and Menopause Clinic, Endocrine and Dermatology Centre, 140 Harley Street, London W1N 1AH (0171 935 2440)

also: § Mr Agarwal, Royal Free Hospital, Pond Street, London NW3 2QG (0181 435 9693)

also: § Mrs M. Hickerton, Balham Health Centre, 120 Bedford Hill, London SW12 (0181 673 1201, appointments, or 0181 672 0317, advice)

also: § Professor Franks, Samaritan Hospital for Women, Marylebone Road, London NW1 5YE (0171 402 4211)

also: § Dr Boutwood, The Bloomsbury Menopause Clinic, Elizabeth Garrett Anderson Hospital for Women, 144 Euston Road, London NW1 (0171 387 2501)

also: # Dr Hubinont, 9A Wilbraham Place, Sloane Street, London SW1X 9AL)0171 730 7928)

also: # Dr Cram, 121 Harley Street, London W1 (0171 935 7111)

also: # Miss Cardozo, 129 Harley Street, London W1 (0171 935 2357)

also: # Dr Dean, 12 Thurloe Street, London SW7 (0171 584 2357)

Macclesfield: § Dr Leslie Batchelor, Well Woman Clinic, Family Planning and Ante-natal Clinic, West Park Hospital, Macclesfield, Cheshire (01625 661169)

Maldon: § The Health Clinic, Wantz Chase, Maldon, Essex (01245 261749)

Manchester: § Mrs Gallimore, Ann Street Health Centre, Ann Street, Denton, Manchester M34 2AS (0161 320 7000)

 also: § Mr Dawe, North Manchester General Hospital, Delauney's Road, Crumpsall, Manchester M8 6RB (0161 795 4567)

 also: § Mrs B. Stevenson, Palatine Centre, 63–65 Palatine Road, Manchester M20 9LJ (0161 434 3555)

 also: § Dr Ann Webb, Wythenshaw Health Care Centre, Stancliff Road, Manchester M22 (0161 437 54625)

 also: § Hope Hospital, Eccles Old Road, Salford M6 8HD (0161 789 7373)

Mexborough: § Mr Genton, Mexborough Montagu Hospital, Adwick Road, Mexborough, South Yorkshire (01709 585171)

Mitcham: # Dr G. Chodbury, Heslemere House, 68 Heslemere Avenue, Mitcham (0181 648 3234)

Moulsham Lodge: § The Health Clinic, Lilac Way, Gloucester Avenue, Moulsham Lodge, Essex (01245 261749)

New Barnet: § Dr Kay, Menopausal and Well Woman Clinic, East Barnet Health Centre, 149 East Barnet Road, New Barnet, Herts EN4 8QZ (0181 440 1251)

Newcastle under Lyme: § Dr O'Brien, 14 Harrowby Drive, Newcastle under Lyme, Staffordshire (01782 614265)

Newcastle upon Tyne: § Dr Roger Francis, Department of Medicine, Newcastle General Hospital, Westgate Road, Newcastle upon Tyne NE4 6BE (0191 273 8811)

 also: # Mr Silverstone, Nuffield Hospital, Jesmond, Newcastle-upon-Tyne (0191 273 8811)

North Cheam: § Priory Crescent Clinic, Priory Crescent, North Cheam, Surrey (0181 685 9922)

 also: * Dr L. Ross, St Anthonys Hospital, London Road, North Cheam (0181 337 6691)

Nottingham: § Dr Filshie, City Hospital, Hucknall Road, Nottingham (01602 691169)

Nuneaton: § Mr M.L. Cox, Gynaecology Out-Patient Department, George Elliot Hospital, College Street, Nuneaton CV10 7DJ (01203 384201 x 22675)

Oldham: § Mr A.M. Mander, The Royal Oldham Hospital, Rochdale Road, Oldham, Lancs OL1 2JH (0161 624 0420)

 also: # Mr A.M. Mander, Lancaster House, 174 Chamber Road, Oldham, Lancs OL8 4BY (0161 652 1227)

Oxford: § Mr D. Barlow, The John Radcliffe Hospital, Headington, Oxford (01865 64711)

Peterborough: § Mr Hackman, Peterborough and District Hospital, Thorpe Road, Peterborough (01733 67451)

Plymouth: § Dr Falconer, Plymouth General Hospital, Freedom Field, Kensington Road, Plymouth PL4 7JJ (01752 668080)

Pontypool: § Dr A. Parker, Gwent Health Authority, Community Health Units, Block B, Caerleon House, Mantilard Park Estate, Pontypool, Gwent NP4 0AX (014955 57911)

Pontrypridd: § Dr D. Pugh, East Glamorgan General Hospital, Church Village, Pontypridd, Mid-Glamorgan (01443 204242)

> *also*: * Amarant Centre at the East Glamorgan General Hospital, Church Village, Pontypridd (01443 218218)

Portsmouth: § Dr Sarah Randall, The Ella Gordon Centre, East Wing, St Mary's Hospital, Portsmouth, Hampshire (01709 548680)

Rochdale: # Mr A.M. Mander, Highfield Private Hospital Place, Manchester Road, Rochdale, Lancs OL11 4LX (01706 55121)

Rotherham: # Mr K.J. Anderton, The Mews, Morthen Hall Lane, Morthen, Rotherham S66 6JL (01709 548680)

Rugby: § Mr L. Harvey, Menopausal Clinic, Hospital of St Cross, Barby Road, Rugby (01788 72831)

Scunthorpe: # Mr Heywood, The Crosby Nursing Home, 207 Fordingham Road, Scunthorpe, South Humberside (01724 721191)

> *also*: § Miss Stringer, The Scunthorpe General Hospital, Cliff Gardens, Scunthorpe, South Yorkshire (01724 282282)

Sheffield: § Dr J. Wordsworth, Central Health Clinic, Mulberry Street, Sheffield S1 2PJ (01742 768885)

> *also*: § Dr Taylor, North General Hospital, Herries Road, Sheffield (01742 434343)

> *also*: § Miss B. Jackson, Sheffield Clinic, 17 North Church Street, Sheffield S1 (017422 768711)

> *also*: § Dr Wordsworth, Royal Hallamshire Hospital, Glossop Road, Sheffield (01742 766222)

Slough: § Dr June Lawson, Menopause Clinic, Slough Family Planning Clinic, Osborne Street, Slough (01753 26875)

Solihull § Mr D. Sturdee, Menopause Clinic, Department of

Obstetrics and Gynaecology, Lode Lane, Solihull B91 2JL (0121 711 4455)

South Woodham Ferrers: § The Health Clinic, Merchant Street, South Woodham Ferrers, Essex (01245 261749)

Stafford: § Mr A.B. Duke, HRT Clinic, Stafford District General Hospital, Western Road, Stafford (01785 57731)

Staines: § Mr P. Saunders, Ashford Hospital, Staines, Middlesex (01784 251188)

Stalybridge: § Mrs Brierley, Stalybridge Clinic, Stamford Street, Stalybridge, Cheshire (0161 338 2728)

Stockport: § Stepping Hill Hospital, Stockport, Cheshire (0161 483 1010)

Stockton-on-Tees: § Mrs W. Francis, Women's Health Advice Centre, 31 Yarm Lane, Stockton-on-Tees, Cleveland (01642 674393)

Stourbridge: § Mrs Widdett (Counselling only), Wordsley Green Health Centre, Lawnsford Road, Wordsley, Stourbridge, West Midlands (01384 271271)

Sunderland: § Mrs Batts, Well Woman Clinic, Pallian Health Centre, Hylton Road, Sunderland (0191 514 4166)

Sutton Coldfield': § Menopausal Counselling Clinic, Good Hope Hospital, Rectory Road, Sutton Coldfield, West Midlands B75 7RR (0121 378 2211)

Sutton: § Mrs J. Groves, Outpatient Dept., Sutton Hospital, Brighton Road, Sutton, Surrey (0121 378 2211)

Swansea: § Dr Anand, Central Clinic (Counselling only), Trinity Building, 21 Orchard Street, Swansea (01792 651791)

> *also*: § Mr P. Bowen-Simpkins (monthly), Gynaecology Department, Singleton Hospital, Sketty, Swansea SA2 8QA (01792 205666)

> *also*: # Mr P. Bowen-Simpkins, 36 Walter Road, Swansea (01792 655600)

Tunbridge Wells: § Family Planning Clinic, 21 Dudley Road, Tunbridge Wells, Kent TN1 1LE (01892 30002)

Uxbridge: § Dr Walefield (Counselling only), Uxbridge Health Centre, George Street, Uxbridge, Middlesex (01895 52461)

Ware: # Mrs Rita Harrison, Health Centre, Bowling Road, Ware, Herts (01920 50705)

Warrington: # Dr Marjorie Monks, Private Care,

(Counselling and Women's) 29 Wilson Pattern Street, War-rington WA1 1PG (01925 50705)

Wednesbury: § Alison Day, Mesty Croft Clinic, Alma Street, Wednesbury, West Midlands (0121 556 0020)

Wendover: § Pat Hancock, Wendover Health Centre, Ayles-bury Road, Wendover, Bucks (01296 623452)

Wimborne: § Dr De Silva (Counselling only), Wimborne Clinic, Rowlands Hill, Wimborne, Dorset BH21 1AR (01202 882405)

Worcester: § Dr Joan Windsor, St John's Clinic, Family and Preventative Care Services Unit, 1 Bromyard Road, Worc-ester WR2 5BS (01905 424979)

Many hospitals which do not run special menopause clinics, and are not, therefore, listed here, will accept menopause and osteoporosis referrals within their obstetric and gynaecology department. In most large hospitals, at least one gynaecolo-gist or endocrinologist has a special interest in HRT. A referral letter is required in all cases under NHS and *preferred* for private consultations with a gynaecologist or at private clinics. If you are seen without GP referral, your doctor will be informed retrospectively. The names of the doctors running the clinics may change from time to time, also some clinics close while others open which means the full accuracy of this list cannot be guaranteed.

Anyone encountering difficulties in obtaining treatment should contact The Amarant Trust, Women's Health Concern or the National Osteoporosis Society, FPA Headquarters, at 27–35 Mortimer Street, London, W1N 7RJ (071 636 7866), will also advise, and can give the name of the nearest meno-pause clinic for any area in the country.

Remember you have the right to ask for a second opinion, or the right to change your doctor, if this should prove neces-sary. You should expect to share in discussion and decisions concerning your health, your body and your bones.

Further reading

The Menopause and HRT
Understanding Osteoporosis, by Wendy Cooper (Arrow, 1990)
The Amarant Book of HRT, by Teresa Gorman and Dr Malcolm Whitehead (Pan, 1989)
The Menopause (A Women's Health Concern Publication, 1985)

Cystitis
Understanding Cystitis, by Angela Kilmartin (Arrow, 1986)
Sexual Cystitis, by Angela Kilmartin (Arrow, 1988)

Nutrition
The Calcium Guide Book (An NOS publication; free to members, £2 to non-members; published annually)
The Dictionary of Nutritional Health, by Adrienne Mayes PhD (Thorsons, 1986)
The Food Factor, (6th edition) by Barbara Griggs (Penguin, 1988)

The Contraceptive Pill
Everything You Need to Know about the Pill, by Wendy Cooper and Dr Tom Smith (Sheldon, 1984)

Hysterectomy
Hysterectomy, by Suzie Hayman (Sheldon, 1986)

Heart and Cardio-vascular Protection
Living with High Blood Pressure, by Dr Tom Smith (Sheldon, 1985)
Living with your Heart, by Dr Tom Smith (Sheldon, 1990)

Index